FEAR2FAITH

FEAR 2 FAITH

Our Journey Through Mesothelioma

Linda Chitwood

To order additional copies of this book, contact:
Xlibris Corporation
1-888-795-4274
www.Xlibris.com
Orders@Xlibris.com
105338

Contents

I dedicate this book to honor the *past* by remembering my witty and absolutely brilliant Mother who died September 28, 2011; to honor the *present* by cherishing every moment with our exuberant and wonderful grandchildren: Jackson, Haleigh, Audrey, and Beau, our newest angel who arrived Dec.7, 2011; and to honor the *future,* by recognizing the untiring efforts of research teams all over the world who are working for a cure for all cancers.

Mom, I miss you each and every day.

Jackson, Haleigh, Audrey and Beau, you are the brightest jewels in our crown of life.

Cancer Research Workers: Never give up working for the cure. You WILL find it.

Jesus said to her, "My daughter, your faith has made you well. Go in peace, and be healed of your trouble."

—Mark 5:34, Good News Bible

Prologue

Faith—the essence of things unseen, the substance of things hoped for. As a Christian, I know that faith is one of the most important components. I know that Christ commands believers to have faith. I know my life is more abundant and full with faith. To be honest, I also know that faith is an area for spiritual growth for me.

Fear—I easily identify fears in my life. I know my response to fear. My heart rate increases, my mouth becomes dry, my shoulders rise, my breathing quickens. I know what fear feels like, yet describing how faith feels is more challenging.

I find fear and faith an interesting dichotomy. Fear is an emotion created for us by God's own hands. I believe fear is useful and needed. However, faith is a belief. Faith is a choice. Faith is God's gift to believers.

This is simply my journey as I traversed the slippery slope of coping with my fear by growing my faith when I found myself reeling with my husband's devastating medical diagnosis of mesothelioma.

I decided to share our story for one purpose—to help others. I am as honest as I can be regarding my emotions, my personal growth, and yes, my journey through along the pathway of faith and fear.

Lannie and I are an average couple. We fell in love, finished our educations, got married, and were blessed to have and raise two beautiful children, Mark and Alison. Our marriage has had its ups and downs, yet we have reached a pleasant sort of peace in our lives. We travel as often as we can, usually to visit family. We are ardent college football fans and have had season tickets at Virginia Tech (VT) since 1998. We are blessed to have educated our children and for all of us to have enjoyed good health.

Our true joy is our wonderful family. Our children are grown and independent. Each of them has children of their own. At the time of Lannie's diagnosis, my son, Mark, and his wife, Jerry, had a beautiful five-month-old baby girl, Haleigh. My daughter, Alison, and her husband, Dan, had a fifteen-month-old adorable son, Jackson, and were expecting their daughter in two months. We adore our grandchildren! We frequently babysit and consider it a joy and a privilege.

Lannie retired in August 2006. He had been a game warden (they are now called conservation officers) in Southampton County for over thirty years. Following his retirement, he became a real estate agent, did some private investigator work, tinkered around the house, hunted and fished to his heart's content, and thoroughly enjoyed being Pee-Paw.

I continued to work full-time. I am a registered nurse (RN), and most of my career has been teaching the art and science of nursing. I have taught nursing for almost thirty years. I provide both classroom teaching and bedside patient care with my students. I am a very hands-on teacher. I also did a lot of home health nursing along the way as a side job to keep my nursing skills fresh and to earn some extra income. I find it immensely satisfying to provide nursing care in a person's own home.

Also, for the first time in almost ten years, my commute to work was less than a fifty-to sixty-minute drive each way. I bade good-bye to traveling the four-lane highway of Highway 460 east or west five days a week. My new job was teaching nursing at a local college (Paul D. Camp Community College), which is only a thirty-minute commute along a scenic country road through rolling farmland countryside. How I appreciated that change after almost thirty-five years of traveling the very busy four lanes of Highway 460! Another bonus was being back at Obici Hospital for the clinical component of the nursing curriculum. It was the new Obici Hospital; the old hospital had been demolished, but it was still familiar to me because I taught many of the nurses still employed there. It was like coming home, in many ways. Life was good, and I was grateful.

Everything was going really well until November 15, 2007.

Part 1: The Diagnosis

November 15, 2007—the first cold finger of fear touches my heart as I listen to his chest through my stethoscope. I should hear even, equal, clear breathing on both sides if all is well. I don't, and my anxiety rises. He has a bad cough and a fever, so I am auscultating his lung sounds. Over the *lub-dub* of his heart rhythm, I hear normal left lung filling and emptying. I hear almost no sounds on the right side. I carefully look him over. His cheeks are pink; his extremities are nice and warm with brisk capillary refill—all indicators of normal circulation. He is not having any difficulty breathing; his heart rate and rhythm are normal. I am an RN with over thirty years of experience, and my nursing mind tells me that these are all indications that he is healthy, not seriously ill. But I feel fear deep within the core of my innermost being. My brain tells me that this instinctive fear is off base, perhaps exaggerated. The instinctive fear remains as I continue to carefully assess him. I tell him he must see Dr. Hall, our primary care physician, tomorrow morning because I am hearing diminished lung sounds on the right side. I am thinking he must have pneumonia. This is very rare for my husband. He has hardly been sick a day in the almost forty years I have known him.

November 16, 2007—It is Friday morning, and even though I have planned an extremely full day of work with my nursing students at the college, I prepare to use a family sick day to go to Dr. Hall's office with him. However, this morning he is feeling fine. He has no fever, he slept well, and his cough is productive. He considers not going to the doctor. I urge him to go, and he reluctantly agrees. He, in turn, urges me to head to the college. We leave at the same time and go toward two different directions. I head for the college with the promise he will call me.

Once I am at the college, I try to concentrate on my work for the day, student oral presentations, but my mind is filled with apprehension. My cell phone is carefully tucked in my pocket and set on vibrate. At 10:10 a.m., it vibrates. I leave the classroom to answer the call. The second cold finger of fear grips my heart as I hear his news: his right lung has collapsed because it is surrounded by fluid and he has pneumonia. He is oxygenating his body with only his left lung and maybe a small portion of his right lung. Dr. Hall wants to hospitalize him immediately to run more tests and to begin IV-antibiotic treatment. He is currently in the emergency department (ED) at Sentara Obici Hospital, awaiting medical-imaging tests and further treatment. Outwardly, I am calm, composed. Inwardly, I am frightened. That cold finger of fear is gaining momentum, encircling my very core. I can feel my heart pounding in my chest, and my mouth is dry. I explain to my students that I need them to finish their presentations as quickly as possible, and I explain why. I reassure myself that it will take time to run the needed medical tests, so I may as well stay and finish the presentations. My heart is not here—I want to be with my husband. At last, the students finish, and I rush from the college to make the twenty-five-mile trip to the hospital, willing myself to drive slowly, safely.

I arrive at Sentara Obici Hospital, this hospital I have learned so well, and go to the ED through the back way. Lannie hasn't told me his ED cubicle number, and I briefly wander only to discover that I don't need the room number because I can follow the familiar sounds of his coughing and easily find him. As I enter his cubicle, I see the fear on his face, and I know my face too mirrors this fear. In an unspoken gesture of a devotion and love born from thirty-two years of marriage, I simply reach out to his hand and gently lay my hand over his. There is nothing to be said. I give him the burger I picked up on the way. Before he can eat it, Dr. Baracat arrives. The third cold finger of fear grips my heart as Dr. Baracat reports that the CT scan reveals three tumors around the lining of his right lung. One is quarter sized, one is nickel sized, and one is dime sized. I amaze myself with the ability to be outwardly calm while I am quaking internally. Tumors? Lannie? A lifelong nonsmoker who was always healthy? Dr. Baracat then performs a thoracentesis—an invasive procedure with a very long needle inserted into Lannie's rib cage to remove fluid that surrounds his affected lung. I am very happy to see Julie, his nurse. I taught Julie many years before, and it is comforting to see her familiar face as she provides assistance during the procedure. I am trying to be brave and in control. Dr. Baracat tells us that the tumors could be only pockets of infection; until a biopsy is performed, it is impossible to know. He tells us about the next steps that will be a surgery called a VATS procedure and a pluerodesis. Even though I am a nurse, I am not familiar with this surgery. I plan a long night on the Internet. This surgery will occur on Monday or Tuesday. Meanwhile, Lannie will remain in the hospital over the weekend to receive IV antibiotics for the pneumonia.

I phone our children, Mark and Alison, with this unexpected news regarding their dad. As our son, Mark, receives the news, he says, "Mom, this doesn't sound too good." I agree. Alison is my more inquisitive child. She and Dan, my son-in-law, are shopping in BJ's when they receive my phone call. Alison responds with a choked voice, "What kind of tumors?" Sadly, I can't tell her because, at this point, no one knows. I try to control my tears for everyone. I don't always succeed.

Lannie and I continue our wait in the ED cubicle. At last, a hospital room is available. Once again I am thankful because it is on the very unit where my students have their clinical experience. Being on this familiar unit brings me comfort. Still, it is very hard to leave him this first night. I want to stay by his side, but I must go home to feed our pets, make phone calls, search the Internet, and try to take this all in.

Saturday, November 17, 2007—morning finds me at Lannie's hospital room bright and early. Dr. Baracat tells us Lannie will have a CT scan of his abdomen and pelvis today. We are both anxious regarding the findings of this CT scan. I have computer access at Obici because I teach nursing students there. This gives me access to Lannie's medical information, including the results of these CT scans. As soon as I determine the radiology reports may be ready for viewing, I check for the results. There are two enlarged lymph nodes in his lower abdomen. Are they the result of his lung infection (pneumonia), which could be normal, or are they are more tumors? I read that the radiologist feels they are most likely malignant tumors. Malignant? I am shocked and horrified at that word. *Malignant.* My mind is whirling like a spinning dervish. Those cold fingers of fear encircling my heart are gripping me forcefully. I take a deep breath and share the findings with Lannie. We calmly discuss all of this. We are both apprehensive. We decide the tumors have to be infection related, not because we are in denial, but because it is the only thing that makes sense. We try to relax and follow our normal home routine for a Saturday afternoon by watching college football games on TV.

We are ardent college football fans, and we had planned to be at the Virginia Tech (VT)-Miami game in Blacksburg today, tailgating with our friends, enjoying the game in our seats at Lane Stadium—until our plans were diverted by this illness. Our game-day tickets lie in his hospital trash can. We tried to give them away, but no one could use them on such short notice. Instead, we are watching the VT-Miami football game on TV. VT wins! I order pizza, and we have a pleasant evening. I search the Internet again when I get home Saturday night. The only thing that keeps popping up is mesothelioma (a.k.a. meso), a usually fatal type of lung cancer that is caused by exposure to asbestos. His doctors have quizzed us thoroughly on asbestos exposure, so I know they are thinking of meso as well. I am sure it could not be meso. He is a retired game warden who worked outdoors all his life. No asbestos exposure that either of us or our children can think of. No, it can't be meso; it has to be infection related.

Sunday, November 18, 2007—I miss church so that I can be with Lannie. Our children and grandchildren visit us in the hospital. Alison is eight months pregnant and is running after her fifteen-month-old toddler, Jackson, who has found a multitude of interesting items in the hospital to be explored! I take him to the lobby and entertain him so everyone can really visit. We are all more positive today. All of us have decided Lannie must just have pockets of infection. It is the only explanation that makes sense.

Monday, November 19, 2007—I am due at Obici early in the morning for another reason: my annual mammogram is scheduled for 8:00 a.m. I had warned Lannie yesterday not to eat any breakfast this morning in case they do the surgery today. I made the necessary work arrangements to have the day off—my coworkers are wonderful. I arrive before my scheduled mammogram to find Lannie wandering around the hospital, trying to locate Dr. McBee (the surgeon) to determine if surgery will happen that day. Following my mammogram, I head straight to Lannie's room. I encounter Dr. McBee dressed in his surgical scrubs standing at the main desk area, reviewing Lannie's chart. He nods to me and follows me to Lannie's room. He explains the procedure and tells us he will operate today, probably before noon.

I am relieved, yet apprehensive. I know this is an invasive surgery. I ask the hospital chaplain to pray with us. I continue fighting fear and apprehension while I try to remain calm for Lannie; I know that he too is frightened. Around 10:00 a.m., we are told the operating room (OR) is ready. I phone our children. Both of them offer to change their plans and come straight to the hospital; we refuse. It is opening day for deer-hunting season, and Mark has been in the woods, hunting for several hours. Alison, a dental hygienist, has a full day of patients scheduled. I am trying to project a confidence to them that I don't really feel—that the surgery will go well and we will get the good news that these "tumors" are just as we thought—pockets of infection. I promise to call them both as soon as I have news. Lannie and I remain together until just prior to his surgery. We are joking with one another, trying to instill calm for each other.

As soon as he goes into the OR, I return to his hospital room to move his belongings to his assigned intensive care unit (ICU) room. Usually, the staff does this, but I do it instead. I need to stay busy, and it takes me about thirty minutes to complete the task. I return to wait in the OR waiting room, and I am there for only fifteen to twenty minutes when I see Dr. McBee walking toward me. He kneels down beside me, looks into my eyes, and says, "The operation went well. He is doing fine. However, I am gravely concerned your husband has lung cancer. I hope that I am wrong. But I don't think I am. I am very concerned that he has cancer." Initially, I remain outwardly composed, calm. Dr. McBee remains beside me for another few minutes and repeats the information. He is kind and caring as he relates this news. I thank him for his honesty and for telling me the truth—I am very thankful for that. My mind is spinning. I feel my heart pounding in my chest, and the sound of my heartbeat roaring in my ears is very rapid. I remain outwardly calm and composed for about eight minutes. I tell myself that I am OK. I tell myself that lots of people have cancer and do well. I tell myself not to panic—that there is no reason to panic. Everything will be OK (whatever OK is).

Then, out of nowhere it seems, a huge swell of emotion surges toward me, and a tsunami of fear, uncertainty, and sorrow submerge me. I feel as though I am drowning, and I can't swim to the top of the wave to fill my lungs with air. Stabbing fingers of fear encircle my core, my being. I finally come to the top of this tidal wave to catch a breath just as tears begin and don't stop. I try to cry quietly; the waiting room is full of families. I fail. A lady sitting close by me offers to get me some water. One of the members of the staff in the waiting room offers me a box of tissues and then asks if I would like her to pray with me. Gratefully, wordlessly, and still softly sobbing, I accept. Our prayer group grows to include two more people: a hospital volunteer and a perfect stranger. We form a huddle as we pray, and I am so very, very comforted by this act of thoughtfulness and the genuine kindness of perfect strangers. I am deeply touched. It helps.

I call my friend and coworker, Carol, to arrange work details for the rest of the week. It is Thanksgiving week, so I only need to cover Tuesday and Wednesday. I continue sobbing softly as I tell her the news. The emotions I have held in check since Friday are pouring out of me. I call Mark. I hear his choked voice telling me he is coming as soon as possible. For some reason, I find myself avoiding calling Alison. I want to break the news to her gently, and I just can't formulate the right words I want to use. Later, I realize it is my protective mothering instinct. She is very pregnant, and I want to shield her from the unwelcome news for as long as I can. Eventually, I call her, and as I tell her the news, I sense that my true feelings are being revealed in the tone of my voice no matter how hard I try to disguise them. She too is on her way to Obici.

She arrives at the OR waiting room, and we sit together. We are tearful at intervals. We talk; we try to make sense of the news. I view her swollen abdomen and ask if she has eaten. "I can't, Mom," she says. "I just can't eat right now." I don't press the matter. She asks me, "What are you going to tell Dad?" I pause. I had not really thought about it. I simply say, "The truth." She nods with agreement.

At last we are told Lannie has been transferred to the ICU. We both go to the ICU family waiting room and continue our waiting there until I receive permission to go to his bedside. His nurse, Kara, is kind and gracious. She senses my desperation to be with Lannie and reunites us while she is still getting him settled—a gesture I truly appreciate because I know it is something many nurses would not do. I look down at his face; his eyes are closed. I hold his hand, a gesture that I sense is mutually comforting. He is attached to many tubes and IV lines. They do not frighten me because of my nursing knowledge. Shortly, he awakens and directly asks me, "What did they find?" I report exactly what was told to me. He exhales deeply and says, "Well, I'm devastated." Dumbly, I nod. I do not cry. We hold hands as we love each other with our eyes. He breaks this moment. He asks for his cell phone; he wants to call his mother and family. I know he needs to do this.

Mark arrives shortly with Jerry and little Haleigh in a stroller. The stress and fear of the situation is etched on his face. Dan and little Jackson also arrive with Dan pushing Jackson in a stroller. The waiting room becomes quite filled with the strollers and our family, but everyone is kind and accommodative. We are all in shock and coping as best we can. Friends arrive. Carol (my coworker and dear friend) brings me a big chocolate chip cookie and a bottle of lemonade. I realize I have had very little to eat all day. I am not really hungry, but it tastes good, and I know I need the nourishment. Carol's thoughtfulness also nourishes my aching heart. She is the first of many visitors who pour in to offer support and care. The outpouring of love and support from my church family, friends, and coworkers genuinely touches my aching heart. It means more than I can ever say.

Other doctors become involved in his care this first afternoon. There are so many unanswered questions at this point. The uncertainty is unnerving, but I give all of the medical team the same message: that we want to know everything, even if it is just a guess at this point. I want them to know that we want to be involved with every aspect. I learn to be careful of what you ask for. Dr. Baracat tells me it is most likely a stage 3 or 4 lung cancer, probably metastasizing from another primary source, most likely the lung or adrenal gland. This cancer cannot be removed from the lung. Wow! This is not the news I had in mind when I asked to know everything.

Until now, I have been holding on to a fragile sliver of hope that his cancer has been caught very early so it can probably be easily removed, treated, and yes, cured. That window of hope has now slammed shut, and panic, born of pure fear, is rising within me. With God's help, I rise above the panic to maintain some sense of control. I am not offended by Dr. Baracat's honesty. Truly, I am appreciative. I know where we stand regarding options. He shows me two pictures of the cancer affecting Lannie's right lung so that I can see why it can't be removed. He lets me keep the pictures, and oddly, they are comforting to me. I share them with Lannie. His cancer looks like little blisters along the lining of his lung. I tell Dr. Baracat that I know a person can live with only one lung, and he quietly nods. My mind is whirling with a million unanswered questions. Our devastating news is spreading. Wonderful friends and family members are calling and visiting. Members from our church family come to the hospital and are supportive, caring. I visit the hospital chapel frequently for respite and to pray—it brings me such comfort. Mercifully, Lannie's surgical pain is well controlled, and his pain medicines soften the reality of the grimness of his prognosis—for a while. I find myself wondering just how much he really understands at this point. I draw strength and comfort from friends, family, and continued prayer.

I leave Lannie on the first night in the ICU under the care of another former student, Susan. I am delighted Susan is his nurse. I know he is in capable hands. I leave Susan my contact information and return home to feed our animals and respond to the many messages on our answering machine. Once home, I am alone with my thoughts and fears. I look at our familiar surroundings. They don't seem so familiar anymore? I begin to realize that everything about our lives has changed with the simple words "I am gravely concerned your husband has lung cancer."

My cell phone battery died on the way home while I was talking with Alison. To top it all off, my eyes are extremely raw and irritated from the combination of wearing my contact lenses during this long, long day and my crying. Somehow, I managed to leave my glasses at home today, so I had to continue wearing my contacts if I wanted to see. I can hardly wait to take the darned things out; if I had known what was ahead of me this day, I would have worn my glasses instead. I surprise myself with a wry smile as I think this. I put my glasses on and head to our computer. I find comfort, perhaps a sense of control, in gathering data. My son-in-law, Dan, is doing the same thing on his computer. Meso is what keeps coming up. I am exhausted and confused. I take a long bath, eat a sandwich, and curl up with Kitty, and somehow, I sleep.

Tuesday, November 20, 2007—I arrive at the hospital at 5:45 a.m. wearing my glasses—no more contact lenses on my irritated eyeballs today! Alison made the very good suggestion that I meet with Dr. McBee again with a list of questions. I am ready with my list. I know he usually arrives at the ICU by 6:00 a.m. He arrives at 6:10 a.m., and he kindly, graciously answers my many questions. He doesn't rush me even though I know he is a very busy doctor. He takes time to answer every question. Yes, he is certain it is cancer. The cell type is clear celled, which makes it look like renal/adrenal cancer. Perhaps it metastasized from the kidney to his right lung? So much uncertainty. I want quick, rapid answers, and I can't have them. Lannie has fared well during the night, and I am grateful for that.

His first cousin (and our dear friend) Elmo, a.k.a. Punkin, arrives from his home in the western part of Virginia that morning. Punkin and Lannie grew up together and, to my eyes, have always seemed more like brothers than cousins. It is so thoughtful and caring of Punkin to rearrange his work schedule and drive several hours to be with us. I am deeply touched. Just seeing Punkin makes me feel better, and I see Lannie visibly brighten and relax as he and Punkin joke and talk. More friends from church visit throughout this long day. I am very appreciative. Mark and Alison and their spouses are all here along with our grandchildren. We huddle, ask questions, and speculate. I try to eat to take care of my body. It is hard. I cry at times. However, now I am wearing my glasses. More doctors come in and give opinions. I appreciate each of them. They have been honest and kind, and I am grateful. Physical therapy comes in, and Lannie gets up from his ICU bed, and he moves well. His mind is still somewhat affected by the pain medicine, and I remain unsure of exactly how much he really understands. I let it go—understanding won't change it. By 7:30 p.m., he is moved out of ICU to a step-down room for this night. I leave around 9:30 p.m. Punkin comes home with me, and I enjoy having him to talk with at home. We have thought of more questions for Dr. McBee, so we plan for another early morning at the hospital.

Wednesday, November 21, 2007—Dr. Forman (partners with Dr. Baracat) takes over for Dr. Baracat. Today I see at once that Lannie is more awake and aware and relates well to Dr. Forman. Dr. Forman and Dr. McBee make rounds at about the same time and answer all our questions. It seems that the cancer is renal/adrenal at this point. That is grim news. I have researched renal/adrenal cancer, and the prognosis is three to eighteen months. I stuff my fear so that I can be strong for my family. But the four cold fingers of fear that envelop my heart remain alive and well, just momentarily contained. Dr. Forman tells me he will have a more reliable diagnosis as to the exact kind of cancer by Saturday. A series of dye procedures on the tissue cells, which take many hours/days, will best help to determine the correct diagnosis. I am to call Dr. Foreman after 5:00 p.m. on Saturday for the news. However, he is certain it is cancer.

With that news, Punkin leaves to return to his home in the mountains, about a four-hour drive. It is now the day before Thanksgiving. He offers to stay with us in Ivor; I encourage him to return home to his family. Lannie is expected to be discharged in the afternoon as well. I keep my mind busy by preparing for that. I try to plan some kind of Thanksgiving holiday for our immediate family. I am painfully, acutely aware it may be Lannie's last. We are discharged around 3:00 p.m. Lannie is irritable and edgy. I am numb and functioning on remote control. He fusses about everything during the thirty-minute drive to Ivor: the traffic, the noise, my driving, etc. My nursing brain kicks in as I realize it is not pain causing his irritability but a reaction to his pain medication. I advise Lannie to avoid taking any more of it; it is time to try another pain medication.

We are home! Our wonderful church family brings us a delicious home-cooked meal. I am so grateful; I have not been to a grocery store for milk, bread, or anything else since last Thursday, almost a full week ago. Thanksgiving is tomorrow, and our church family is also bringing us Thanksgiving dinner. I am moved to fresh tears with their thoughtfulness and generosity. Once we eat, Lannie and I finally talk about the cancer. We discuss his symptoms, and we both cannot imagine it could be renal/adrenal—he has no symptoms of it. We say few words; our eyes communicate in the unspoken way of a couple who have been together for many years. There is not much to say; at this point, we are simply coping—together. We find comfort in each other. At last, we tumble into bed after this exhausting day. I am careful of his incision sites and pain level during the night, but I am glad he is beside me.

Thursday, November 22, 2007—Thanksgiving Day finds Lannie up and about early and moving well. He looks so incredibly healthy that the events of the past few days seem like a bad dream. I try to sleep in; I am exhausted, but peace of mind evades me. I try to absorb that Lannie may be dying, that I might be a widow by this time next year. I feel incredibly saddened. My sadness motivates me to get up, get dressed, put on a brave face, and get through this day. Our family will have our Thanksgiving dinner tomorrow along with my son-in-law's parents, Jack and Agnes. I like Jack and Agnes, and I look forward to seeing them.

Our church brings our wonderful dinner, but more importantly, they visit for a while. Susan, one of the meal deliverers, is a recent breast cancer survivor who also visited us in the hospital and encouraged us with her story. She and Lannie joke, and she lifts our spirits. Lannie and I discuss her case, and he feels optimistic. I wonder again how much he understands of the prognosis, so I ask. He tells me he wants to wait until the test results on Saturday. I agree, and at last, we go to bed together. I remain careful of his incision sites as I snuggle next to him.

Friday, November 23, 2007—as planned, we have our family Thanksgiving. It is good to have people here. Lannie is uncharacteristically irritable at times; I blame the remaining pain medicine. Our children notice it too. His irritability is taken in stride as we visit, laugh, and enjoy our time together. I am truly thankful.

Saturday, November 24, 2007—the day to call Dr. Forman arrives. Lannie is soundly sleeping on the sofa at 5:01 p.m. I call, and Dr. Forman answers immediately; I know he is expecting my call. He tells me it looks like renal/adrenal cancer from the pathology reports at this point. He tells me more testing (dyes of the cells) is needed to be conclusive, but it is clear celled, which looks like renal/adrenal cancer. My heart sinks, and I am harshly reacquainted with those very cold fingers of fear enveloping my heart as Dr. Forman softly adds, "Linda, this is going to be very difficult to treat, very difficult." I clearly understand his carefully veiled message. In a choked voice, I thank him for his honesty. I consider waking Lannie to tell him the news; I decide against it. He is so tired. He is still recovering from major surgery; he is sleeping so well. It is the wrong decision. When he awakens at 5:48 p.m., he asks the results, and as I tell him, he is furious that I did not awaken him so that he could talk with Dr. Forman. Fortunately, I am able to reach Dr. Forman immediately, and he and Lannie talk. After that conversation, Lannie and I talk and set boundaries regarding information sharing. I am aware that my desire to protect him must have limits, and I respect that. I think Lannie begins to understand some of the burden I have been carrying, and we both understand each other better. Our children have already called to find out the test results; we call other friends and family. I feel shocked (again), almost numb. Lannie is already on the Internet, exploring renal/adrenal cancer, but he stops shortly; the information is just too devastating. I continue Lannie's search, and it *is* depressing—very. However, Lannie has no symptoms of renal/adrenal cancer. It is not denial, but I truly question the diagnosis as I absorb the changes in my life for the last nine days.

Sunday, November 25, 2007—our family attends church. We are surrounded by caring friends. Their support and devotion to Lannie and to us raises my spirit. It is at this precise moment that I find myself beginning my second phase of this journey of adjusting to life with cancer. I will myself to let go of the burden of fear I am carrying and give it to God through Jesus Christ so that I can feel some measure of peace. I try my best to have faith—faith that all will somehow be right again, whatever that is. Mostly, I feel confused, overwhelmed, and still scared, yet I sense that God, with His infinite grace that I will never deserve, understands me. With just that tiny bit of faith, I feel some measure of peace.

Monday-Tuesday, November 26-27, 2007—I return to work for portions of the day. It is nearing the end of the semester, and I have a heavy workload that must be completed. Lannie is still weak and recovering from the surgery and needs me at home. He has CT scans, PET scans, and many doctor visits scheduled in the next weeks, and my mind swirls as I try to figure a way to go with him to each one and still complete all my work at the college. The end of the semester means even more tasks and less flexibility. My students, coworkers, and boss are flexible and wonderful, and that brings me strength.

Wednesday, November 28, 2007—my last week of clinical for the semester arrives. I go to clinical early Wednesday morning to the very unit in which Lannie was so recently hospitalized. The staff kindly inquires about him and us. I still feel numb and answer politely, "He's OK." How do I explain the shock of absorbing that my previously wholly healthy husband is now fighting terminal cancer?

Dr. Forman arrives to the unit and seeks me out. He tells me that he has been checking Lannie's pathology slides daily and that his slides are now looking less like renal/adrenal cancer and more like mesothelioma. This news literally stops me in my tracks, completely. I stare intently at Dr. Forman. My gut tells me that this is the correct diagnosis—I am certain of it. For the first time in almost two weeks, I feel a tiny ember of hope flickering in my heart. The ember is there just flickering, sputtering in my chest, and I fear my excitement at this unexpected news may extinguish it! If Lannie has meso, there is a very risky surgery that he can undergo that may help him. I have read about it, and I know it is risky, dangerous, and difficult. But it is a chance at life, and that alone sustains this tiny ember of hope I am beginning to feel.

I break my own clinical rule (about using the phone during clinical hours) and quickly call Lannie, Mark, and Alison with the news. The tiny ember of hope I am feeling is also felt by them; I sense it. Maybe, maybe, there is something besides the certainty of terminal cancer in the picture now. It is not lost on any of us that meso is also a deadly cancer. I know of no one who has survived it. However, it is simply the lesser of two evils, and at this point, we are thankful for that. The next few weeks are a blur.

November 29-December 18, 2007—we continue the rounds of doctor visits, CT scans, PET scans. His cancer continues to look more and more to be meso. Lannie also has an appointment with wonderful Dr. Su, who is one of the best hematologists/oncologists I know. During our appointment, Dr. Su is very honest and doesn't mince words. Meso is deadly. The only hope of surviving it is the risky operation I have read about called an extrapleural pneumonectomy (EPP). EPP involves the removal of Lannie's cancerous lung, the lining around the lung, the lining around his heart, half his diaphragm, and one rib. It is a very risky surgery, and surgeons will only perform this operation if the meso is caught early—in stage 1 or early stage 2. If the cancer is stage 3 or 4, it is simply too late for the benefits to outweigh the risk of the surgery. This is significant for us because of those two lymph nodes that are showing up suspiciously in his abdomen. They could be a result of the recent pneumonia, or they could be metastasis of the meso that will put him in at least a stage 2, maybe stage 3. Dr. Su tells us that doctors will not perform the surgery if Lannie's meso is determined to be stage 3. As I hear this news, fear, my constant companion, once again rises above my suppression. However, my fear is momentarily delayed as I interpret Lannie's facial expression and body language while he absorbs this latest news. I can see he is struggling mightily.

He tells Dr. Su, "I really don't want to lose my lung." Who can blame him? Dr. Su answers again that the EPP is the only hope, and it is a small one at that. I know he is correct because I too have researched

EPP. Dr. Su tells us that currently, chemo and radiation bring only palliation (relief of symptoms) for anyone with meso to enhance quality of life for a few years. Lannie continues to assimilate this awful news. He asks how long he will live if he chooses not to have the surgery. Dr. Su says eighteen months to three years. Dr. Su adds that life with meso is difficult, painful at times. I am looking anxiously at Lannie. It is his decision to make. I sense and understand his hesitation at the thought of this incredibly invasive, devastating surgery. I feel so utterly helpless as I watch him grapple with this tough, tough decision. I can see he is digesting this information. After a moment, Lannie straightens his shoulders and looks up directly at Dr. Su and asks, "How old are you?" Dr. Su replies, "Sixty-two." Lannie then asks, "Would you let them take your lung?" Without a moment's hesitation, Dr. Su answers, "Yes."

God bless Dr. Su. With that answer, Lannie quietly nods his head affirmatively. My heart is breaking as I watch this brave decision unfold. Dr. Su offers to help us with admission to any hospital or cancer center. He mentions Duke, Johns Hopkins, other famous centers. We thank him, and I promise to communicate with him regarding our decision. On the way home, I call our children with the latest news. I break down as I relate the information—not because the news is unexpected, but because I am so touched by Lannie's bravery during this tough decision. It is a cold, dark, and rainy December night. Lannie is driving back to Ivor. My tears blur the image of the rain pouring down from the darkened sky as it hits the windshield. During this thirty-minute drive home and in the cocoon of our rain-enclosed car with only dim lights reflecting from other vehicles, I pray. I pray for God to lead us to the treatment center to which He would have us to go. I pray for strength to face the battle ahead. I pray for a measure of peace to enter our hearts.

By the time we arrive at our doorstep, I feel a measure of peace. I concentrate on what we have to be thankful for. I realize I am thankful for our competent doctors and nurses. I realize we are blessed to even have the option of the EPP. That ever-present ember of faith is glowing, and I feel my fear recede. I face Lannie and share these thoughts with him. I see his eyes light up, his shoulders square, and his fighting spirit return. God is so good. Faith is here.

The next few weeks continue the flurry of medical tests, decisions, continued prayer, and ups and downs. The ups: Dr. Forman found a surgeon, Dr. Harpole, who performs the EPP surgery at Duke University Medical Center, and he made the arrangements for us to go for an evaluation on December 18. I know this is an answer to one of my many prayers; I am so thankful. The downs: Dr. Harpole requires a PET scan that our insurance initially declines to cover. I am furious, heartsick at the knowledge that a doctor employed by the insurance company, who knows nothing about Lannie's case, can make this kind of decision. I furiously fight the insurance company tooth and nail. Fortunately, Dr. Forman knows how to work with the insurance company, and with Dr. Su's help also, the test is finally covered by our health insurance plan. However, the results of the PET scan were frightening. The two hot spots in his abdomen remain suspicious, and the radiologist feels they are most likely a metastasis. Ugh. Does this mean that the cancer is a stage 3 or 4 and that Dr. Harpole will not be able to perform the surgery, which is our only hope? The taste of fear once again rises like bile in my throat. However, the ups continue to show: God places many cancer survivors in our path who had devastating prognoses, yet they survive. Their stories inspire me and feed my flickering flame of faith.

Another up is that Lannie and I became friends with another couple in nearby Matthews County who have experienced meso and the EPP at Duke University Medical Center. Their names are Dave and Becky. Their daughter worked with my sister in nearby Gloucester, and the two of them arranged for all of us to talk via the telephone. Dave's case is very similar to Lannie's. Dave had always been healthy, and suddenly at age fifty-eight, he developed pneumonia. Eventually, he was diagnosed with meso and was also offered the EPP. His surgeon was Dr. D'Minco, not Dr. Harpole, but all his surgery was performed at Duke. They spend well over an hour with us during this first phone call; we have so many questions. God bless Dave and Becky; they patiently answer every question of what I am sure is not a pleasant experience to remember.

Dave is doing well, and their story fills us with hope. I am very aware that every case of meso is unique, but we both feel hope as we talk with this wonderful couple. Dave and Becky share details of their personal research regarding meso, give me some resources to check, and offer lots of support. Lannie is very direct while speaking with Dave. Two of the initial questions Lannie asked Dave are the following: "Can you breathe all right now?" and "Could you breathe when you came out of the surgery?" I have known that the breathing issue is a big hurdle for Lannie, understandably so. I see him visibly relax as he hears Dave's affirmative response that, yes, he breathes OK now and he was able to breathe on his own immediately following the EPP surgery. They also offer us practical information regarding parking, hotels, and the like. They have three grown children that are close to the ages of Mark and Alison. As Becky and I get to know each other better, we share "mom" and "wife" stories in that unique way of two women who share an unspoken yet very real bond. My admiration and appreciation for both her and Dave grow. They are a huge blessing to us. I am thankful.

As the months of November and December roll along, I discover one more surprising aspect of our new life of coping with cancer. Ironically, it is that daily life, with all its challenges and joys, continues as always. Bills must be paid, jobs completed, commitments fulfilled, and our summer vacation must be planned. So during the hectic months of this November and December, Alison finds herself contemplating our annual family vacation that usually takes place at Cape Hatteras sometime during the summer months. In past years, she is the one who finds a cottage large enough to accommodate the families. Ideally, it is best to reserve a cottage by December. Usually, she narrows the cottage search to five to six possibilities, and then we, as a family, thoroughly study and discuss the merits of each cottage following our Thanksgiving dinner. We then finalize the reservation in early December. However, this Thanksgiving, we didn't even go there. Meanwhile, Alison found a wonderful cottage and called to ask me about planning our usual Cape Hatteras vacation. Her question momentarily catches me off guard. I am stumped. Vacation? Sometime in the *future*? I hesitate. I am unsure of what to say. Then from somewhere, an electric surge of fierce determination and positive power courses through me. I feel warm, strong and, for the first time in weeks, certain. Without another moment of hesitation, I tell her to reserve that cottage for our usual week. We *will* have our family vacation. We *will* have the joy of planning and looking forward to it. I feel a calm peace envelop my psyche as soon as I make the decision. Immediately I call my mother with this news of our planned summer vacation. My mother's response is every bit as positive. "Yes," she says, "absolutely. Of course we will go to Cape Hatteras just as we always have!" This one simple gesture of planning our summer vacation fills me with an apprehensive sort of joy. I am only too aware that planning a vacation for this summer is quite a risk. That's OK. For reasons I can't really explain, I feel that I have scored a victory over cancer with my decision, and it feels *great*!

I also continue to be thankful for every blessing in our lives. Our church continues their loving support. Our friends and families continue their prayers. Alison's pregnancy, with the promise of new life, continues smoothly. I focus on the ups—most of the time.

Part 2: The Surgery

Monday, December 17, 2007—our appointment at Duke is for tomorrow at 9:00 a.m., but we are planning to leave our home sometime this afternoon. Early this morning, I give my last exam at the college. I finish all the paperwork involved and turn in my grades and reports for the past semester before noon so that I can return home as soon as possible. We leave Ivor at 2:00 p.m. It is only a three-hour drive from our home in Ivor, but we have chosen to spend the night in Durham so that we won't risk any chance of a delay for tomorrow. As we head to Durham, I am once again amazed at how deceptively healthy Lannie looks. He is only one month out of a very invasive surgery, yet his color is pink. He moves easily, no signs of lingering incisional pain, no shortness of breath. My mind wanders briefly—could this really be happening? Are we really headed to Duke in hope that Dr. Harpole would say yes to removing Lannie's right lung? We arrive and check into our hotel room.

We spend a fitful night. I don't think either of us sleeps much. However, faith is currently winning the battle over fear in my heart for one main reason: In the weeks (has it only been four weeks?) since Lannie's diagnosis, my dear friend Tracey (she also is an RN. We attend church together, and she was one of our first visitors at Obici after Lannie's VATS and pleurodesis surgery) sent me a wonderful, encouraging, and empathetic letter I cherish. I reread it numerous times as fear continues its assault on my overwhelmed psyche. Tracey and her husband, Kenneth, are very special friends to me. They were baptized at the same time as our son and Ken and I were ordained together as Deacons. Our lives here in this small, close knit community, have intertwined in many ways. Tracey and Ken have faced their own battles with chronic illness because their daughter Kelly Anne has cystic fibrosis. During one of Kelly Anne's hospitalizations, Tracey was studying her Bible and was led to Matthew 9:19-22. It is the Bible verse about the woman with a chronic bleeding issue who reached out to touch Christ's cloak with the faith that if she just touched Christ's cloak, she would be healed. Jesus knew He had been touched and turned and saw her touching His cloak. Jesus tells her that she is healed, that her faith has made her well. This Bible verse greatly comforted Tracey, and she wanted to share that comfort with me, so she wrote me this thoughtful letter to share her experience. I have read and studied that passage many, many times. However, now it has a different meaning to me.

As I try to relax on this evening, I find myself again contemplating the mystery of faith. Does it have to be a mystery? Does my human limitation make it a mystery? Does my desire for concrete answers mean I lack faith? Many questions fill my mind and intrigue me.

For about twenty years now, my nightly Bible devotional consists of reading a selection from *The Upper Room*. In our hotel room tonight, with the anxiety of Lannie's appointment with Dr. Harpole looming in front of us, I pull out my Bible with *The Upper Room* carefully tucked inside it. My mind is filled with a myriad of questions concerning "what ifs" regarding tomorrow's appointment. The biggest "what if?" is: What if Lannie's cancer is a Stage 3 or Stage 4 and he isn't a candidate for the EPP, which is his only hope to fight the meso? I ready my mind for my devotional by trying to empty my mind of anxiety so that I can truly concentrate on His Word. At last I feel ready to begin reading, and what do I find? Tonight's reading is from Mark 5:24-34, which is Mark's account of the woman with the bleeding disorder. I am certain that the timing of this verse is a true message from God sent directly to comfort me. I concentrate on faith, not fear. It helps.

Tuesday, December 18, 2007—the first of many tests to my newly determined faith occurs the next morning. As we prepare for our visit with Dr. Harpole, Lannie takes his morning shower. During his shower, a segment comes on CNN regarding a man who dies from mesothelioma. I watch as his wife describes his painful death in excruciating detail. My heart sinks as I identify too closely with the pain etched on this woman's face. Momentarily, I succumb to despair, then I tell myself that *I will have faith*. I never share the news story with Lannie.

We arrive at the Morris Cancer Treatment Center promptly at 8:55 a.m. As we enter the waiting room area, I am absolutely amazed, astounded at the sheer volume of people who are here to be seen. We wait in line to be registered. We wait again for lab tests. We wait again to be called for Dr. Harpole. While we wait, I observe others. With some couples, it is easy to determine the caregiver from the patient. With others, I cannot easily distinguish the roles. I find myself wondering about each person's circumstance. Everyone is friendly. A few engage us in conversation as we share "war stories". The sharing of stories helps to pass the time and lowers my apprehension. My mind wanders. What if Lannie's mesothelioma is too far advanced to get the surgery? What will be our options? Quietly, I take a deep breath to quell my fear with faith.

Everyone here speaks confidently about the quality of care at Duke; I am thankful to be here.

At last, Lannie's name is called. Our first meeting is with a resident. He examines Lannie as Lannie repeats his now-so-familiar story to this new doctor. The resident is calm, interested. He asks Lannie, "What is your understanding of what the surgery can do for you?"; a good open-ended question. Lannie responds, "The surgery should get most of the meso, and then radiation and chemo will get what is left behind." The resident hastens to clarify that meso is difficult to treat and that meso has a poor prognosis and other bits of negative information before I interrupt him and say, "We know this. We have done our research. This surgery is our only chance. It is our only hope." Quietly, reflectively, this doctor nods his head.

We go to a different exam room. Initially, there is an unsettling quiet between Lannie and me. We have been harshly reacquainted with the glaring reality of the meso diagnosis and prognosis and the uncertainty that Lannie will qualify for the EPP. Lannie breaks the silence with an attempt at a joke. "Well, at least he didn't say I was too far gone to get the surgery." I manage a weak smile. Neither of us speaks much; we are on edge as we wait for Dr. Harpole. A soft knock at the door introduces Dr. Harpole with the same resident following him. I recognize Dr. Harpole from his picture on his website. Dr. Harpole carries a palpable energy, intensity, a welcome sense of enthusiasm, and certainty for his work. I instantly sense his intelligence, his passion, and his sense of positive energy. My spirit lifts. I look at Lannie, and I see the same feeling reflected on his face. Dr. Harpole's positive energy revives our flagging spirits. He examines Lannie and hears his story. At last, we hear the words we long to hear. "Let's look at when we will plan the surgery." With those words, he takes a felt-tipped pen and begins to draw the proposed incision line on Lannie's chest. I catch Lannie's eyes for just a moment as Dr. Harpole moves around the exam room. Lannie's blue eyes are now bright with hope. Seeing Lannie's hope revives me, and I feel the ember of hope that dwells within my heart swell and burn brightly too.

Dr. Harpole explains the necessary steps for the surgery. First, we need a definite diagnosis of mesothelioma. Lannie's diagnosis is still somewhat questionable; Duke wants to perform their own pathology testing to be certain. The danger of the EPP surgery is such that certain protocols are required to validate the meso diagnosis. We make arrangements to have Lannie's pathology slides transferred from Obici's lab to Duke's lab for further evaluation. A tentative surgery date is set for January 10, 2008. I mention to Dr. Harpole that our daughter's due date for our expected granddaughter is January 20. He offers to postpone the surgery until after the baby's birth, but Lannie adamantly refuses with an instant response. "I want this devil out of me!" I assure all of us (especially myself) that with God's help, we will manage both the birth and surgery. Alison plans to be present for the surgery, so Dr. Harpole tells me that if Alison should go in labor while at Duke with Lannie, he will contact his wife's obstetrician for the delivery. I smile. I am touched by his thoughtful, helpful gesture.

However, Dr. Harpole feels certain the cancer is meso, so we go ahead and finalize plans for the surgery. We are to return on January 8 for the confirmation that Duke agrees with the certainty of the meso diagnosis, and then we will complete the rest of the preoperative workup: blood tests, EKG, CT scans, etc. I hesitantly ask about the two hot spots on the PET scan. Dr. Harpole shakes his head and tells me, "I'm not too worried about them. Meso doesn't go there usually. We will watch them." I nod my head with relief because I know Dr. Harpole is a meso expert, and I have confidence in what he says. The pre-op workup is scheduled for January 8. I mentally calculate my college work schedule. The new semester (and my teaching responsibilities) begins January 7.

Oh well, just another detail to be worked out. I ask Dr. Harpole his best guess of how long Lannie will be in the hospital following the surgery. He hesitates briefly and says seven to ten days but hastens to add that it may be less or more. I understand. I remember that our friend, Dave, was in the hospital about ten days for his EPP. I ask how long Lannie will be on a ventilator. For some reason, the thought of Lannie on a ventilator unnerves me. As a nurse, I know a ventilator will probably be necessary, at least initially. Dr. Harpole pauses and carefully considers his answer. "He may not need to go on one. Let's wait and see."

Before we leave, we make all the necessary appointments and hotel arrangements for the proposed surgery. We tour some of the Duke campus while we walk back to our car. It is a cool, cloudy day, and the Duke campus is pretty, well maintained, clean. I notice that Lannie walks so easily, no shortness of breath, and he has a nice pink color. I can't help but wonder how much all of that will change with one lung, instead of two, to oxygenate his body. Dr. Harpole has told Lannie to exercise by walking all he can between now and the surgery. It is the middle of deer-hunting season, so this is music to Lannie's ears. He can hunt deer all he wants and complete his walking requirement. We leave Duke with lighter hearts and a small but strong sense of optimism—a welcome change. More than anything, we feel a sense of humbleness. We are only too aware that we could have left with little or no hope.

We call our families with the news. I also begin to think about the Christmas holiday—I have done little to prepare for it, and it is December 18. I have not even sent the first Christmas card. I usually have my cards in the mail, with a little family newsletter, by the first week in December. Until now, I didn't know what to include in the newsletter. So as I am riding back home, I mentally compose the newsletter and organize activities for Christmas. It helps me. I refuse to think that this may be Lannie's last Christmas, and I am determined to stay positive, and I do.

Medical bills are arriving four to five at a time every day. I have good insurance with my job, but the co-pays are significant. I am trying to save every penny I can because I know I will be staying in a hotel and eating out for ten to fourteen days with Lannie's surgery, plus the price of gas, parking each day he is in the hospital, etc. His medicines are expensive also. I push all these concerns away; I will simply pay what I can.

We have a wonderful, simple, family-oriented Christmas. I find myself deeply appreciative for the simple pleasures of the season. A sweet smile, a caring word, a pretty wreath, the joy of watching our grandchildren's excitement—these joys are deep and satisfying and enough.

I start a new semester, with all its joys and challenges, at the college on Monday, January 7, 2008. We leave for Lannie's pre-op workup early in the morning on January 8. Once again, we arrive at Duke and wait to get registered, wait for the lab tests, and then wait to see the doctors. At last, we see Dr. Harpole, and he smiles as he tells us that the cancer is definitely a clear-celled meso and that the surgery is scheduled for the day after tomorrow (January 10). We are relieved—it is our hope for survival. Dr. Harpole explains the procedure, risks, expected recovery, and the grueling postoperative course, which includes intense radiation and chemotherapy. He does not paint a pretty picture at all. At one point, he predicts, "You won't like me too much by this summer." Lannie looks briefly to me before he issues his retort. "Bring it on. I am ready to get this stuff out of me!" We ask more questions, and at one point, Lannie dares to ask about the possibility of truly being cured from this awful disease. Before answering this loaded question, Dr. Harpole pauses briefly then looks directly, intently into our eyes and tells us with fierce determination, "I want to eradicate it. That is my goal." My heart lifts as I hear these words, and at this moment, I realize, really realize, that practicing medicine involves healing someone's inner heart as much as their outer body. I have new respect for this gifted surgeon.

We spend the rest of January 8 completing a vast array of medical tests and signing what seems to be a never-ending plethora of papers. It is during the signing of one of these many papers that a most profound story is revealed to us regarding Dr. Harpole and a former patient. A lovely lady in a crisp white lab coat arrives from the Duke research team. She explains to us that one of the papers requiring Lannie's signature is asking for permission from him to donate his diseased lung and other organs (that would be removed during the surgery) so that they can be studied with the hope others would benefit. Since one of my many prayers is that somehow God will use us and this experience to help someone else and to lessen their burden, Lannie signs with no hesitancy. I share my prayer and our desire to help others with this lovely lady. Thoughtfully she listens, and I sense she is weighing something in her mind before she responds to us. After just a moment's hesitation, she says, "Since you feel this way, I want to share this story with you."

This is the story: Dr. Harpole was scheduled to perform lung surgery on a lady who was somewhat apprehensive regarding her proposed surgery. At some point during the preoperative visit with Dr. Harpole, she said to him, "Dr. Harpole, before I let you operate on me, I want you to do something first." Dr. Harpole agreed. She then stood up and said to Dr. Harpole, "Stand up." He did so. She said, "Place your hands in mine." He again complied. As she held his hands in her hands, she looked him in the eye and slowly asked, "I want to know one thing before I let you cut on me. Are you a man of God?" Never breaking the hand hold or the eye contact, Dr. Harpole responded with these simple words, "His hands guide my hands." With that, the apprehensive lady was satisfied and continued with the planned surgery. My heart lifts as I hear this story. I feel a profound sense of peace pour through my heart and mind. It inspires and comforts me. How I embrace this welcome sense of peace; peace of mind has been a rare experience since his diagnosis. More than all of Dr. Harpole's many notable accomplishments and accolades, the simple words "His hands guide my hands" mean the most to me. I am so thankful this lady cared enough to share it with us.

We are told to call tomorrow after 4:00 p.m. to learn the surgery time. Dr. Harpole tells us the surgery will last anywhere from six to ten hours. We have a three-hour trip from Ivor to Durham, so we plan on leaving Ivor around 4:00 p.m. tomorrow; I will call early and hope they have the surgery time. We hit the road for home, knowing that we will be returning down these same roads in less than twenty-four hours for surgery that will forever alter our lives.

We call family and friends with the latest news regarding the planned surgery. I tell my daughter about the story of the apprehensive patient and about Dr. Harpole's fierce, determined response regarding eradicating the meso. She excitedly interrupts me. "Mom, those are the exact words I have used while I have been praying. I have prayed that God would guide Dr. Harpole'shands and that he would eradiate Dad's cancer." I am amazed at God's grace for us at this moment. I know this lovely lady and her willingness to share this remarkable story is a gift from Him. I am grateful.

We are both guardedly optimistic while we ride home. I realize I must finish packing for a possible two-week stay as well as prepare for the class I am teaching tomorrow as soon as I get home. Our very expectant daughter (her original induction date was to be on January 11, the day after tomorrow.) will ride with us to Duke tomorrow, and she is bringing her OB records as well as an infant car seat and clothes for the baby should she deliver our granddaughter at Duke. Our son will follow in a different car. I contemplate a million details as I try to organize all that I must accomplish in the next twenty hours. As long as I keep my mind busy, I can keep myself from dwelling on the seriousness of the surgery.

During the ride home, one cold finger of fear reaches but does not grip my heart. I actively fight it. I concentrate on God's blessings to us: a competent, caring medical and nursing team; my good health; the promise of a soon-to-be-born granddaughter; a loving circle of family and friends—too many blessings to count. Our church has surprised us with a love offering of money to help us with expenses. Words can never convey my surprise and appreciation for this thoughtfulness. Also, Tracey, my dear friend, created a beautiful "comfort basket" loaded with all sorts of useful items and comfort foods for us to take to sustain us at Duke. My coworkers remain flexible and supportive as I navigate the conflicting paths of devotion to my family and commitment to my job. Two ladies in our church have agreed to stand in for me and be with Alison and Dan during the birth if I am unable to be there. Of course, I desperately want to be present for the birth, and I actively pray for that to happen, but I must be prepared should that not happen. At last, we pull into our driveway for a very short stay.

Wednesday, January 9, 2008—morning brings a change of mood for both of us. I feel heavy and somber as I prepare for work. We are both up very early. Lannie plans early visits with our two grandchildren, eighteen-month-old Jackson and six-month-old Haleigh. I can see that the reality regarding the seriousness of this difficult surgery is weighing heavily on his mind. It is the same for me. I am finishing the last of the packing before I leave for my workday at the college; we need to leave for Duke right at 4:00 p.m. It keeps my mind occupied.

During the drive to work, my mind has time to absorb all that is ahead of us. I am overcome by overwhelming anxiety, and I just break down. I pull off the road, and I cry for a while. Eventually, I pull myself together, drive to the college, and by God's grace, teach my first class. Then during a class break, I get a phone call from Lannie. His voice breaks as he says, "I just had to say good-bye to Little Man [Jackson's nickname]." I hear the anguish in his voice—I can only imagine how wrenching this is for him. Lannie so cherishes and so enjoys our precious, wonderful grandchildren. Of course, I know he is wondering if this good-bye will be final. He is on his way to see Haleigh now. We talk. Once again, I feel so helpless because I know there is little I can say. Words offer little comfort.

After I finish that phone call, I break down again and sob quietly in my office. My dear friend and coworker, Amy, comes in and offers kindness and caring. I am so upset that I feel ill, nauseous. By His grace, I pull myself together and teach my last class. God gives me the strength to do this, and somehow, I do. Yes, I could have asked another faculty member to teach either of these classes, but it is my responsibility, and I feel the need to do it. At last I head for home. It is a warm, sunshine-filled January afternoon. As I arrive, I see Lannie walking around the perimeter of our large yard, taking it all in, saying good-bye, I think. My heart wrenches at this sight. I walk out to greet him, and silently, we embrace. There are no words.

I wait until 3:30 p.m. before I call for the surgery time. The surgery time is set for 12:00 noon, and they want us to be at the hospital by 10:00

a.m. I give my contact information should there be any change. We call our Duke support team: wonderful Punkin; Punkin's sister, Judy (Judy and Punkin are first cousins to Lannie); and her husband, Frank, to tell them the proposed time for the surgery. They live about ninety minutes from Duke. I am particularly grateful to have such a strong support team when we are three hours from home. Our home church has only an interim pastor right now. He offered to come, and several members from our church offered to come as well, which is so thoughtful of them. We settled for prayers from home instead. It is very comforting to know that these good people are with us in thought and prayer. We all agree to meet in the Duke main lobby at 10:00 a.m. Shortly, Alison arrives at our house, complete with a suitcase for the baby and the infant car seat. Mark arrives shortly after that. We project a feeling of confidence and security once we are all together. We plan the itinerary for the trip to Durham and leave Ivor right at 4:00 p.m. We stop for gas and supper around 5:30 p.m., and my cell phone rings. Duke is changing his surgery time from 12:00 noon to 1:30 p.m. They want us to arrive at the hospital by 11:00. Ugh—the last thing I want is to have to sit around waiting for this surgery with our anxiety mounting. We call our support team with that news; we all agree to stick to our original plan and to meet at 10:00 a.m. in the lobby anyway.

We arrive in Durham at our hotel around 8:00 p.m. and check in. We are sharing a suite with a large bedroom with two queen-sized beds and a living room with a sofa sleeper and mini-kitchen and two bathrooms. Mark takes the sofa. Alison will get one bed, and Lannie and I will take the other. The four of us are in a strange sort of humorous mood where we are actively trying to find humor in anything. I guess it is a type of dark humor to protect us and help us cope with our anxiety over the impending surgery. We talk and joke. Lannie has composed an informal will of sorts—to whom he wants to leave his hunting/fishing stuff, his truck, etc. We joke and tell him, "You're not pushing up daisies in the Ivor cemetery yet!" We *do* find humor, and I have never been more proud of my tough, good-hearted family. We are in this together. Lannie and I have already signed the documents for advanced directives, and I understand and will follow his wishes regarding resuscitative measures. He has given me power of attorney should he be unable to make decisions. These are difficult things to contemplate and to discuss, but we did them with a matter-of-fact attitude. The surgery is that risky. At last, we have a group prayer, and then we all go to bed.

In the soft light coming from the lamp beside my bed, I follow my usual nighttime ritual as I read my Bible verse from *The Upper Room. I can hardly believe what my eyes are reading.* Once again, it is the passage regarding the woman with the bleeding issue whose faith heals her. Unexpectedly, my eyes fill with tears. What comfort these familiar words bring to my anxious heart! I reread it. I know, absolutely know, this is a message from God sent directly to me. Concentrating on faith, at last, I fall asleep.

I awaken very early in the morning. I can see only darkness from the gap between the hotel room's curtain and the windowsill; I can't see the clock to know the exact time. Lannie and I are sleeping "spoon style" with my body curled against his back, my arm draped over his chest. I feel the movement of his chest with his breathing. His breathing is even and unlabored. I wonder, *How will his chest movement change when he only has one lung to breathe? How will his chest feel to my hands with one of his ribs gone? What will his incision scar be like? What will life be like after this surgery?*

I rise up on one elbow carefully—I do not want to waken him or Mark or Alison—to look at him. He is so very handsome. He looks so deceptively healthy. His color is pink; his dark-blond hair is thick and shiny resting against the white pillowcase. His shoulders and chest are muscular and broad. I feel the strength of the muscles in his right arm. What will happen to this man I love during the next twelve hours? I actively fight fear. With strength that comes from God, I practice self-control I never had before, and I remain calm and focused. I know that if I show my fear, it is harder for my family. In the darkened twilight, I pray. I pray for God to guide Dr. Harpole's hands and mind. I pray for the anesthesiologists and the nurses. I pray for strength for each of us. I pray for us to stay calm and focused. I pray for the health of our unborn granddaughter safely cocooned in our daughter's uterus. Our son-in-law, Dan, is traveling from Chesapeake, Virginia, later today with little Jackson. Mark's wife, Jerry, is arriving from their home in Wakefield, Virginia, with little Haleigh tomorrow. I pray for their safety and safe travel. I pray for my faith to grow. Lastly, I pray to accept God's will for the outcome of this surgery.

Thursday, January 10, 2008—dawn brings bright sunshine and moderate temperature. I throw some comfort items in a canvas tote bag that I will keep with me all day—it will be a long day at the hospital for all of us. I manage to eat yogurt for breakfast and encourage Alison to do the same. It is hard to eat. The cold, grim reality of the day is hitting all of us—hard. Our mood is tense and we are all anxious, but we are trying to be positive as we cope with our feelings. We arrive at the Duke parking garage around 9:45 a.m. and meet and greet our support team in the lobby as planned. Amid the chaos of activity of the busy lobby, my cell phone suddenly rings. It is the Duke Hospital Surgical Center. "Where are you?" they ask me. I reply, "In the lobby of Duke Hospital." "Good," they say, "because Lannie's surgery time has been changed, and they are ready for him now." They give me instructions on where to go, whom to see, etc. My heart is racing as I relay this news. I see the change in all our demeanors with this welcomed but unexpected change. I am trembling. Lannie is outwardly calm; his hands are cold as ice. The next hour is a whirlwind of activity. We register at the surgical center. We meet different members of the surgical team and relay information. We joke some. Punkin keeps the atmosphere light but caring. I am so thankful for him. Judy is kind and caring. Frank is supportive. Lannie changes into his surgical gown. We join hands as Frank, a retired pastor, prays. I draw great comfort from this prayer, and I feel a sense of peace.

Mark, Alison, and I follow Lannie's stretcher to the pre-op holding area. Although many hospitals allow one family member to stay with their loved one in the pre-op holding room, at Duke, the holding area is usually off-limits to families. During his pre-op workup, I specifically asked about going in there to be with Lannie for as long as possible prior to the operation. I was told that our family would be able to stay together with Lannie for a few minutes. However, a young nurse sees us enter and tries to stop us at the door with the words, "You can't be in here." I curtly reply, "We are leaving in a moment." She persists and follows us, saying, "You are not supposed to be back here." I nod and again assure her that we will be out shortly. We meet his anesthesiologist, and we immediately like him. He is a pulmonary anesthesiologist. I sense his intelligence and level of caring. He motions for us to ignore this nurse and hides us behind the curtain. He answers all our questions. Yes, this is a really big surgery. Yes, it will take many hours, so don't panic if the surgery goes on for a long time. Yes, this is one of the biggest surgeries they (Duke) do. Yes, Lannie should do well because he is otherwise healthy. Yes, he will be with Lannie until it is over. Yes, he may be on a ventilator when he recovers from the surgery. With one last hug and kiss from each of us to Lannie, we leave. I refuse to think that this may be the last time our lips ever meet; I do anyway.

As we prepare to settle in the lobby for The Wait, I sense Mark is troubled. Mark looks to me and says, "Mom, I want to see Dad one more time." I never hesitate. He and I immediately head for the pre-op holding area again and enter as the door swings open to let someone exit. The same young nurse spies us as we try to sneak in—uh-oh. She remembers us and pounces quickly. "I told you. You cannot be in here." I nod my head to her and say in my sweetest, most sarcastic tone, "Sure—be right out in a minute." Quite frankly, unless she has a stick of dynamite hidden in her pocket, she is not going to stop my son from seeing his dad at this moment. Period. The anesthesiologist also remembers us and is actively beckoning us back to Lannie. We visit one more time, and after Mark makes himself satisfied, we leave. On the way out, a different nurse with a kindhearted smile and a friendly expression stops us. She has witnessed the whole exchange with the young nurse and tells us, "I wish I had been the one to see you first. I would have let you spend all the time you wanted with him." I give her a quick hug—how sweet of her!

We are given a communication device; it is similar to the vibrating disc that many restaurants use to communicate when your table is ready. We are told that it will vibrate when they have news for us regarding

Lannie. We begin the wait. I will myself to remain upbeat, positive. I am a nurse. I have an idea of what is proceeding with Lannie through the closed doors of the OR suite. I assess Alison's swollen, very pregnant abdomen. We walk. We call our church family. We call our friends and biological families. Knowing others are praying for us is immensely comforting. We eat lunch while babysitting our communication disc. The surgery is supposed to begin around noon, and they are supposed to call us once the surgery has begun. I surprise myself and actually eat lunch. I force myself to eat a little more than I want. I know it will be a long while before I eat again today, and besides, if Alison sees me eating, she will eat more, which will be better for the baby. I am still a mom! Punkin and Frank keep Mark occupied. Judy sits with me and Alison, and we engage in "women talk"—marriage, pregnancy, children, etc. I keep watching the communication disc. It hasn't moved. We return to the waiting area. At 2:00 p.m., I am antsy. I go to the desk person and tell him that I think our disc is broken since it hasn't moved. He clicks at his computer and tells me that the surgery is in progress and that the incision time was 1:01 p.m. I nod and relay the news. Gradually, the afternoon passes. I try to read; I can't concentrate. I actively pray for the surgical team and Lannie's stamina.

Judy is a sensitive, strong communicator who keeps me going through this long afternoon. We are indoors, but I can see the sun is starting to descend as I look out of the waiting area window. It is just past 5:00 p.m. Our communication disc still hasn't moved; I remain convinced it is broken. As I approach the same desk clerk to inquire about Lannie, I am interrupted by Dr. Harpole himself, dressed in full surgical garb. My heart lurches as soon as I see him. Before he can speak, I hurriedly ask, "Can I go to get everyone?" I want everyone in our support team to hear the same report and have the opportunity to ask questions. He nods, and I quickly gather everyone. We sit in a private area as Dr. Harpole gives us good news. Lannie came through the surgery. He tells us about the amount of blood Lannie lost and that it is being replaced with transfusions. He also tells us, "I got it" (meaning the cancer). I know this is a figure of speech; only the pathology report can confirm the extent of the cancer. However, I know that Dr. Harpole is a meso expert, and I take heart with the notion that he feels he got it. He answers more questions and tells us what to expect over the next twenty-four hours. He will keep Lannie very "dry"—decreasing his fluids to prevent fluids from overloading his remaining fragile lung. He shows us the ICU where Lannie will be taken within the next hour or two to recover. I give him a big hug as he leaves, and then I almost fall apart. I feel the familiar tidal wave of emotion pour over me. I manage to whisper hoarsely, "Thank you, God. Oh, thank you, God." The intensity of my voice startles me. I feel battered and bruised from the stress of this day. More than anything, I *am* so very thankful.

I am also feeling a desperate need to visualize Lannie now that the surgery is over. I wonder if he is on a ventilator—I forgot to ask Dr. Harpole that question. I sense that Mark and Alison feel the need as well. The three of us—along with Punkin, Frank, and Judy—discuss strategies to see him as he is being wheeled from the OR suite. Another patient's family member overhears our planning and tells us that Lannie will come down one of two hallways. We immediately stake out each hallway and wait. The first stretcher comes carrying a male patient, but it is not Lannie. We wait again. The next patient is Lannie, and the anesthesiologist we met earlier is pushing the stretcher. Quickly, I notice that the anesthesiologist is not "bagging" Lannie (which would mean Lannie is not breathing on his own and needs to have the bag fill his lung with air). Lannie is breathing on his own—without the use of a ventilator. This is great! Relief washes over me. The anesthesiologist recognizes us and waves to us, and we yell to Lannie, "We love you! You made it! We will see you as soon as they let us!" I know Lannie hears us because he gives a weak thumbs-up. The anesthesiologist smiles and motions for us to wait. We wait while he settles Lannie into the ICU. He eventually comes out and tells more about the surgery. Lannie is breathing well on his own with the one lung. He then advises that we go eat some supper. It will be a while before Lannie is stable enough for even a brief visit with us. I offer a prayer of thanks, once again, for this wonderful medical and nursing team.

Dan has arrived with little Jackson. Jackson's energetic presence lifts our spirits as he toddles around the ICU waiting room, investigating every nook and cranny. He is a welcome reminder of life and joy. We head to the dining area, and I try to eat. For some reason, I am feeling very fragile and emotional right now. I am fighting back tears and I don't know why. I focus on my family and Judy's caring presence. Judy has a gift for knowing just exactly what to say and do to bring comfort to others. Once again, I realize I am so glad she and Frank are with us this day. We take our time eating; we know that the earliest we will get to see Lannie will be around 7:00 p.m. I so long to see him and touch him. I am always impatient, and this particular wait is especially difficult, even though I understand why. I focus on precious little Jackson—the best therapy for me.

At last, it is after 7:00 p.m., and we head back to the ICU waiting room. We wait a little longer, and we are finally allowed a short visit with him. My heart is racing with anticipation as we approach Lannie's ICU cubicle. Lannie is hooked up to a plethora of tubes and lines. Again, I am not intimidated by them because of my nursing knowledge, but these tubes represent a harsh reminder of the fragility of Lannie's condition. He sees us first and whispers hoarsely to us, "I can breathe! I can breathe!" I hear the note of triumph in his voice. He looks at Frank (who has a short stature) and asks, "Why don't you stand up, Frank?" and then laughs at his own joke. We all laugh too, especially Frank. I know it is important for Lannie to show us he can make a joke. His nurse comes in to tell me that Lannie is her only patient tonight. I sense she knows that I am a nurse too even though I haven't told her so. I leave her my cell phone number and beg her to call me if they need me for anything. We say our good-byes to Lannie, and I kiss his lips and smooth his hair. "I'll see you first thing tomorrow morning," I promise him. I assure him that I am only a phone call away and that the nurse has my number. He nods and looks at me with tired eyes. It is incredibly hard for me to leave him; I so want to remain by his side. We both understand, without speaking it, that it is best for me to go. I kiss his forehead again; we each say our good-byes and leave.

We make plans for tomorrow. Our support group wants to return to be with us; God bless them. I know they are exhausted, and they have over an hour to drive to their home in Rocky Mount, North Carolina. I thank them for everything they have done for us today, and I mean every word of it. I wonder how I could have made it through this trying day without their presence. They have been so wonderful. It is then that Franks amazes me by saying, "Linda, you have each been a blessing to us. Being here with you today has been our blessing." I know he means every word, and I am deeply moved by this wonderful and gracious couple and family. I hug each of them one last time before we all leave.

Back at the hotel room, we are all tired but, once again, humorous. Jackson is toddling about, investigating every inch of the hotel suite that he can reach. We share different things that have happened to us this day and our different perspectives. Alison has a wonderful mind for details and remembers things the doctors told us that, I guess, I didn't hear. Mark shares with me that he has been texting (a skill I have not yet acquired) family and friends with Lannie's progress all day. Somehow, we bathe Jackson, take showers, and ready ourselves for bed. Then Mark surprises me—he comes in from his sleep sofa and requests a group/family prayer. I am touched and so proud of him. Mark is tough on the outside, yet so kind and caring on the inside. His dad's cancer has been tough for him. Jackson is asleep in the Pack 'n Play, so quietly, Dan, Alison, Mark, and I join hands, and I pray thanksgiving for God's abundant mercy and kindness. We all sleep.

Part 3: The Recovery

Friday, January 11, 2008—we arrive at Duke the next morning to find Lannie sitting (his bed folds to a sitting position). He looks pretty rough to my practiced eye. However, it is completely understandable; he has endured a terrible surgery. I meet his nurse. She is friendly, efficient, and knowledgeable and answers my many questions. Lannie's pain is OK, but he is nauseous, probably a side effect of the pain medicine. He is putting out minimal urine, and I ask about that. Dr. Harpole wants to keep him as dry as possible. Lannie is licking his dry lips; he is thirsty but understands he can't have any fluids yet. Lannie tells me he almost passed out when he was put in a sitting position earlier this morning. I can see the experience frightened him. His nurse hastens to explain that it happened because his fluid volume is being purposely kept low (dry) to protect his lung. I understand, and I reassure Lannie. Dr. Harpole comes by while I am there and removes the NG tube (the tube that goes through his nose to his stomach) and explains again why he is keeping him so dry. I trust Dr. Harpole. Lannie asks him, "When do you think I can have something to drink?" Lannie's dry lips and thirst are not lost on Dr. Harpole. He allows the nurse to offer Lannie some foam swabs to dip into water to moisten his dry lips and mouth. Initially, Lannie just moistens them. However, it is not long before he begins to dip them in the water and slurp all the moisture he can gain from them. His nurse and I estimate he is not getting too much, and he continues to slurp to relieve his thirst. All things considered, he is fairly comfortable and doing well. Dr. Harpole is pleased with his progress and tells me, "He is exactly where I want him to be." I am thankful.

The ICU only allows a few visitors at a time, so we go in tag teams so that everyone in our support team can spend time with him today. Ever vigilant, I watch to make sure he is not getting too tired. His nurse is very generous in allowing my visitations, and I express my appreciation. "Actually, I am glad you are here," she replies. "I am assigned to your husband and one other patient, and he is supposed to be my sicker patient, but the other patient has been taking a lot of my time. I am glad you are in here with him." I smile my appreciation to her. About 2:00 p.m., I notice a change in Lannie's EKG. I am not a cardiac nurse, but

I know his rhythm reading is not normal. His nurse enters and looks at his monitor too. Before either of us speaks, the ICU doctor comes in (Duke staffs this ICU with a doctor 24-7) and tells us that she is certain this is a normal variation of Lannie's heart adjusting to his pericardium (lining around his heart) being removed, but she is ordering tests to validate that assumption. The tests later reveal she is correct, but it is a scary time and another unwelcome reminder of the seriousness of this surgery.

Mark's wife, Jerry, and baby girl, Haleigh, arrive safely in the afternoon. Our support team has grown! We take up a large portion of the waiting room; no one seems to mind. We meet other ICU families. Everyone is friendly and shares helpful information gleaned from long hours of waiting. We learn that we can get discount parking tickets. We also learn which nurses are sticklers for following the visitation rules and which ones are more generous.

Lannie is faring well, all things considered. His pain is controlled. His oxygen levels are good, and he is as comfortable as possible (except for the thirst issue). Dr. Harpole visits again this evening and reassures us of Lannie's good progress. He speaks of moving him to the step-down unit this evening, but there are no empty beds available. I am relieved. I want him to stay in ICU at least one more night and day because there is an MD right in the unit 24-7 and the nurse/patient ratio is better. Tonight, I remain at the ICU by Lannie's side while our children, their spouses, and our grandchildren are back at the hotel. The little ones are tired, and Alison is fully nine months pregnant and needs her rest. I plan to leave around 9:00 p.m. It seems it will be easier for me to leave Lannie now; I hope that the wrench that grips my gut as I leave won't be as forceful now. I like to think that we are both adjusting. His evening nurse is pleasant and caring. Once again, I hug Punkin, Judy, and Frank good-bye. I urge them to stay home tomorrow if they wish; however, all three of them assure me they are returning tomorrow. I am so glad. Their support and presence has uplifted and encouraged me. I leave my cell phone number with Lannie's nurse and write it down in several conspicuous places in his ICU room. When the moment comes for me to leave, once again I struggle. It is still hard to leave him. His fatigue makes it easier for me; I can see he needs to rest.

Saturday, January 12, 2008—morning arrives with bright sunshine. For the first time in days (or is it weeks?), I am actually hungry. We make a quick stop for breakfast and get to the hospital by 9:00 a.m. Lannie looks better. His neck pain (probably from the position he was in for the surgery) is worse. Dr. Harpole is allowing some fluids, but to my practiced eye, I can see that he is just "well" enough to begin to really feel the effects of this surgery. He looks dazed, tired, but lights up when one of us enters his room. His nurse today tells me that as soon as a bed is available in the step-down unit, he will transfer there. I stay with him most of the day as I trade visits with our children and their spouses. Trying to contain an active seventeen-month-old toddler in a hospital setting is a challenge. We manage. Haleigh is still in a stroller, so she is a little easier to manage. By afternoon, I am alone with Lannie as the grandchildren need naps and everyone else has returned to the hotel room. He lets down his guard a little; I ask him how he really feels. "Very tired," he responds. It is enough said. I hold his right hand as we both rest.

A room is available around 3:00 p.m. He "graduates" to the step-down unit as planned, and we meet his new nurse. She is young, friendly, and caring. She notices the VT sweatshirt I am wearing and tells me she graduated from Liberty University in nearby Lynchburg, Virginia. I like her friendliness; I can see Lannie does too. His neck is still hurting badly, and the move has taken its toll on him. He is walking slowly, but I am thankful he is walking. Our family arrives, and he is reunited with his precious grandbabies. He is happy to see them, but we all sense his overwhelming fatigue. We make arrangements for me to stay until 10:00 p.m. Alison will return for me then. I marvel at her; she is fully nine months pregnant and running after an active toddler as well as being there for her dad.

Lannie and I share a quiet dinner in the fading light of this cold January night. He is allowed a restricted diet now. I eat my sandwich with him while we watch TV. Eating together while watching TV, a simple pleasure I have always taken for granted—until now. We walk the hall triangle slowly and carefully. Lannie shares what he remembers from the surgery, which isn't too much. I share with him how we passed the time while we waited. I look at him and say, "You know, we are very blessed. God has been so good." Quietly, he nods. We know. He sleeps off and on until 10:00 p.m. I kiss him good-bye on the lips and assure him I will be there early tomorrow morning. I want to be there to meet with Dr. Harpole.

As I pray that night, I reflect on the past few days. I am so acutely aware of the fragility of life and God's grace. I view Alison's unborn baby girl in her womb, and I know He is gracing us immeasurably. I am a planner; I like to organize activities. I now realize that planning gives me only a pseudo sense of control. The events of the past few months have taught me many lessons—all of them valuable, but certainly not always welcomed. Mostly, I am so very grateful for such little things: the simple pleasure of holding Lannie's hand, the enjoyment of a shared meal. Jackson and Haleigh's sweet little smiles and their boundless energy and enthusiasm for exploring life fill my soul with joy. I am so very grateful for competent doctors and caring nurses. I am so appreciative of the support from our many friends. I am so very proud of my children's strength and dignity. I am so very appreciative of my wonderful son-in-law and daughter-in-law for their love, support, and care.

I awaken sometime very early in the morning. It is still dark outside the curtained window. Alison is softly twisting about in her bed beside Dan. Jackson is in his Pack 'n Play, sleeping soundly. She quiets briefly and begins moving again. I watch this pattern for what I am sure is well over an hour. Is she in labor? We have come prepared. Just as I decide that she must be in labor, she falls back to sleep, as eventually I do. Later I discover she was definitely having contractions every five minutes. They just stopped on their own. My feeling of thankfulness increases.

Sunday, January 13, 2008—Dr. Harpole gives us a good report. Lannie is progressing well. He can eat real food later today. Lannie looks better. His color is pink; his oxygenation levels for his body are good. His neck pain is improving, and his pain control is effective. I can honestly say I am amazed. I share with him the news of Alison's contractions during the night. "Well," he says, "let's have that baby!"

The morning is spent with our children, their spouses, and our grandchildren. It is a little crowded, but everyone is sensitive to the effect of so many visitors on Lannie. A group of friends visit and bring my mother-in-law. I can see that she is overwhelmed by all the tubes and machines attached to her son. I can only imagine how hard it is to see your son of fifty-eight years look so vulnerable. We all eat lunch together in the hospital cafeteria. I try to answer her questions and be supportive for her, but I struggle. The events of the past few days have left me feeling vulnerable. Our children are leaving shortly to make the four-hour trip back to their homes. I feel a real sense of loss at their leaving. For the past four days, we have been sharing the hotel room(s), and I realize just how much I enjoyed returning to discuss the day's events and Lannie's progress. Often, they saw or noticed something I missed. I am really going to miss their keen observations. I kiss them all good-bye, pray for their safe return, and return to Lannie's hospital room.

My mother-in-law and that group of visitors leave, and other visitors arrive. Their arrival is welcome, but I am concerned that Lannie tires easily. I worry about offending them if they have to leave so soon after driving several hours to get here, but everyone is understanding and takes their cue without offense—one more of God's many blessings. I think of my wonderful church family back in Ivor. I know that we were lifted up in prayer today during the worship service. I miss them and that fellowship, but I feel uplifted by their prayers.

Lannie continues to walk around the triangle. He actually logs a full mile! I remain thankful, grateful. Our children return safely home as well. I stay until about 9:30 p.m. and leave my cell phone number with his evening nurse. I kiss him good-bye and promise to be there early in the morning. The hotel room is lonely, empty without Jackson eagerly exploring every inch of it. I bathe and again reflect. My cell phone is almost dead; I have been updating everyone with Lannie's progress. The comfort basket from Tracey with all sorts of good comfort food in it—herbal tea, healthy snacks, Nabs, candy bars, etc.—is a welcome sight. Until tonight, I have been too preoccupied to really explore the contents of the comfort basket. Now, with the cold January night just outside the hotel room door, I sip on a cup of hot tea and indulge myself with some delicious munchies. No wonder it is called comfort food! I feel my body and mind relax for the first time in days. I read from the book of Proverbs in my bible and I find peace.

Monday, January 14, 2008—I arrive at the hospital by 7:15 a.m. His night nurse tells me that Lannie had a fairly restful night. He looks OK to me. Dr. Harpole makes his rounds and tells us that he may go home as early as Wednesday. I look at Lannie as we digest this surprising news, and I see immediately that his feelings mirror mine: joy that he is doing so well that he can go home, fear at the thought of being three hours from this safe environment. Still, we nod as we hear this news. It is then that I really begin to think about our future. What does it hold for us? I feel that familiar sense of fear trying to encircle my heart.

Two members of our church family, Joy and Randal Branch, arrive around 9:00 a.m. It is so good to see them. Thoughtfully, Joy has prepared homemade chicken soup for us to warm in the microwave, along with all needed utensils and bowls. Their support really lifts me and lessens my anxiety. They take me to lunch; it is nice to be away from Lannie's hospital room for even a little while, yet I feel I must return to him quickly. I discover that I really don't need to return quickly. He is just fine; it is just that "feeling." Following their wonderful visit, Randal offers a brief prayer, and he and Joy leave. I am so thankful for their visit.

The remainder of the day finds Lannie is in good spirits. He logs many miles around the triangle. His pain is well controlled, and his color is good. He asks me stay and spend the night with him at the hospital tonight. Briefly, I consider staying. I hate to leave him if he really needs me . . . Eventually, I decide it is best for me to return to the hotel room.

Even though all I have really done is I sit beside Lannie, or help him walk around the triangle, or just care for him, I feel exhausted. I know I need to take care of myself, or I will not be able to give my best to him. I am torn. His night nurse is the same young lady from last night. I know she is very competent and familiar with his case, and that comforts me. Still, I hesitate and consider staying. However, she urges me to return to the hotel room. Eventually, Lannie concurs that I need my rest and should return. Once again, I leave my cell phone number with her with strict instructions to call me if Lannie needs anything. Lannie is peaceful and resting when I leave around 10:15 p.m.

Back at the hotel room, I take a quick shower. It is very cold outside. I have just settled in to watch the local news when my cell phone rings. Lannie is on the phone and tells me that he has had a bad reaction to his pain medicine. He is disoriented and frightened. My hair is still wet and I am in my pajamas, but I am already dressing to return to the hospital as I am talking with Lannie on the phone. I tell him I am coming, but his nurse intervenes and tells me that she has the situation under control. Lannie is oriented now and sitting at the nurse's station with her. She assures me that all his vital signs and his oxygen levels are OK. She assures me she will call me if Lannie needs me. She encourages me to stay at the hotel room and get my much-needed rest. Lannie also encourages me to remain at the hotel, so I stay. I prepare to arrive at the hospital early the next morning.

Tuesday, January 15, 2008—Dr. Harpole changes Lannie's pain medications but tells us that pain control is likely to become a challenge since he has had the reaction to the narcotic. He really needs the narcotic to control his pain, yet the reaction he had is cause to discontinue that medication. We take a "wait and see" approach.

This morning brings more visitors from my wonderful church family: my dear friends Tracey Stallard (the "Bible verse and comfort basket" friend), Nancy Stephenson, and Betsy Cutwright. I am close with all these ladies, and their visit means so much to me. Once again we all go to lunch, and Lannie seems to be faring OK with the change in his pain medication. Tracey is an RN, and we discuss pain management strategies from the nursing viewpoint. Nancy offers a prayer before they leave, and I lift Lannie up to God once more as we continue this recovery. However, shortly after our friends leave, I see Lannie's pain level rise visibly. I know that the effects of the narcotic are gone, and the non-narcotic pain medicine isn't effective. He tries to walk the triangle, but it just hurts too badly. I have a long talk with his nurse and advocate finding a solution for effective pain management. I will accept nothing less. She is receptive and caring and obtains an order for one dose of morphine. Lannie gets the morphine and, within an hour, is experiencing some relief. It is not total relief, but it is enough that he is not in severe, agonizing pain. I am grateful for that.

He tries again to walk the triangle; it is very hard. Dr. Harpole arrives for rounds and is immediately concerned about the pain-management issue. He makes some medication changes, and we hope for the best. He tells us to plan on being discharged tomorrow. I am very concerned about pain management for the three-hour trip home. I request for Lannie to receive an IV pain medication "to go" for the trip home. I also have lists of questions for Dr. Harpole: How will I know if Lannie is having a lung infection? How many times per hour is it normal for him to cough? What are the signs of respiratory distress with only one lung? How am I to manage his pain? What foods can he eat? How much walking is enough? What about weather extremes? We have five steps (stairs) up to our house: will climbing five stairs be too much for him? My mind is flying and, to top that off, tomorrow's weather forecast is for snow and ice. My anxiety level is high, and those old familiar fingers of fear are trying to encircle my heart.

Dr. Harpole pleasantly, patiently answers my questions. He then summons Lannie's case manager; she answers most of my questions and calms some of my anxiety. I remain somewhat troubled; there are so many unknowns. My nursing mind wants strict parameters and guidelines, and I realize there aren't very many. I feel the full weight of responsibility for Lannie's care bearing down on me as I return to the hotel room that night. I feel heavy, burdened, and overwhelmed. I read my Bible and once again find the scripture verse comforting. I pray for God to lessen my fear, to sharpen my mind for the important changes in Lannie's condition, to bring his pain under control, and to bring us safely home. I pray for my daughter and unborn granddaughter; her induction date is Friday, and I so want to be, need to be, with our daughter for the birth. I lift all this up to God and pray for His divine healing for this entire situation. I do my best to listen for God's message, and I feel an immediate sense of peace. I realize that I am a good nurse with very strong assessment skills. I feel certain I will recognize any significant changes in Lannie's condition and respond appropriately. I feel a sense of confidence in myself and the situation. I feel certain that, with God's help, I will cope. Immediately the phone rings; it is my son. He has arranged to have Friday off so that he can stay with Lannie, which means that I can be with Alison for the birth. I take a deep breath and feel my anxiety lessen. At last, I fall asleep.

Wednesday, January 16, 2008—morning finds me at the hospital very early. I do not want to miss Dr. Harpole's early morning rounds. Yes, Lannie is being discharged home today! I am thankful, yet apprehensive, tense, and anxious despite last night's brief respite. I bombard the case manager with more questions, especially regarding pain control. I continue my campaign for Lannie to receive a bolus of IV pain medication "to go" for the three-hour drive home. I look at him, and all I can think is that he has practically been cut in half and somewhat pieced back together with internal sutures and external staples. I do not want him to suffer unduly with all the bumps and jiggles in the car during the long trip home. Initially, there is some hesitation regarding my requested pain medication—mostly related to the timing and details of his discharge. Someone works out the details, and eventually, I am assured he will receive the IV pain medication "to go".

My other questions regarding his postoperative home care are answered, some more completely than others. I am feeling the full weight of responsibility for caring for my husband who is still so medically fragile. Am I up to the task? This surgery is so invasive and so radical that, yes, it frightens me to be so far from Duke. His incision is huge—even to my nurse eyes. It begins just under his right shoulder blade and continues to just under his right breast. It is healing well but is a stirring visual reminder of the seriousness of the surgery. I take a deep breath, concentrating on my nursing ability and God's faithfulness throughout this entire ordeal. I have faith He will continue to guide me if I just let Him.

I leave Lannie midmorning to finish packing our car, check out of the hotel, fill his many prescriptions, and eat an early lunch. I feel apprehensive and concerned. I organize and plan every detail of the discharge I can think of. I plan to fill his prescriptions in North Carolina first, even though this means that I will have to have the prescriptions transferred to our local pharmacy after we return to Ivor. I want to have all his medicine available and ready should he need it.

I prepare a bed for him in the front passenger seat of our large Buick, complete with a pillow and the famous soft "blue blanket." The blue blanket is legendary in our family—we all want it when we are sick. It is just a soft warm thermal blanket, but there is just something about it that is so comforting. I know Lannie will need all the comfort I can arrange for the three-hour trip home. I return to the hospital to coordinate the discharge, and at about 2:00 p.m., after he has received his IV pain medication "to go", we leave Duke University Medical Center to head for Ivor. Lannie is reclined on the large front seat of the Buick, the blue blanket snuggled around his shoulders, his soft pillow nestled under his head. He is as comfortable as I can make him. We leave Duke University Medical Center.

The trip home is, thankfully, uneventful. It is cool and gray outside; the snow and ice forecast for today is now expected tomorrow. The old Buick lumbers down the road while I anxiously watch Lannie from the corner of my eye. He sleeps most of the way. His color is pink; his pain is fairly well controlled—for a short while. In Emporia (two hours into the trip and one hour from Ivor), he complains of surgical pain. I give him appropriate medication and I offer him fluids, and we are on the road again.

After the stop in Emporia, I find myself reflecting while I drive the final hour of the trip. Many of the emotions that I have suppressed this last week are rising, invading my consciousness. For the first time, I realize that while I am so very thankful for Lannie's survival through this surgery, I do feel an aching sadness and a painful sense of loss as well. Immediately I feel guilty; I should be so thankful that he is doing so well, and I truly am very thankful. Yet if I am being honest with myself, I acutely feel a sense of loss as well. Suddenly, with blinding clarity, I realize that I am truly grieving the loss of Lannie's health. I am startled at the impact. It is a humbling realization. I have so taken his good health for granted all these years. Lannie has always been so strong, robust, and healthy. I never ever even questioned his strength or health status prior to making plans because it was never an issue. Yes, I am so grateful we are returning home from this massive surgery, but I know our lives are forever changed by cancer. I can't even fathom radiation and chemotherapy, yet I know both are right around the corner. I contemplate all these things as I drive toward home.

I edge closer and closer to our home. On the way, I pass the road that turns off to our church, and I am unexpectedly hit with an emotional meltdown. Where in the world are these feelings coming from? While Lannie sleeps, I can't stop the tears, and for once, I don't try to hold them back. What a relief to just let them go! What a relief to not have to pretend I am strong and to just be able to let the healing power of the cleansing tears just happen. Why am I emotional now? I guess part of the answer is that these familiar roads home are so very comforting—like putting on my "comfy" clothes after working in tight, constrictive clothing all day. Perhaps this comfort level is greater than my well-used defenses. Has it really been only six days since we were headed in the opposite direction, filled with uncertainty about the outcome of the surgery? None of this is lost on me as home grows closer. My reflecting time yields these personal insights: I am humbled. I am grateful. I have changed and grown emotionally and spiritually.

I continue my assessment of Lannie's condition, and it seems to me that even though he is sleeping soundly, he senses home is near. He has slept almost the entire three-hour trip back to Ivor, yet now I see a definite change in his breathing pattern and body position. He is moving about stiffly, awkwardly, in the confines of the Buick's front seat. As I turn left to enter our driveway, Lannie stirs from his makeshift bed and stiffly tries to sit up. I am driving very slowly as he looks around at our driveway and our house. He looks to me, and I know he sees my tears, but he doesn't seem surprised or ask me why. Once we are fully stopped in our driveway, he slowly sits up all the way. He continues his perusal of our surroundings by looking out of the Buick's windows for a few more minutes. I sense he is taking it all in. I sit and watch him. He continues just looking. It is cool and gray in Ivor, and our yard's grass is winter brown; the trees are bare of foliage. He studies it all for just a few more moments; I can see he is in deep thought, and I do not intrude. However, our big Black Lab, Jake, is not so patient! Typical of that unspoken bond between dogs and their owners, Jake, too, senses Lannie's mood and is doing his best to wait. He is anxiously sitting right outside Lannie's car door, looking up at him through the car window as he vigorously wags his tail in a fanning motion against the driveway pavement to welcome him. Jake is actively making his "glad" sound. Definitely, Jake is man's best friend! Lannie nods to Jake, smiles, and turns to meet my eyes. As our eyes meet in that unspoken way of a couple who communicate without always speaking, I realize that he is carefully considering that just one week ago, he was questioning whether he would ever return here. My eyes, locked on his, affirm understanding of his unspoken message. It has only been a few moments, but I sense he has found the peace he has been seeking.

Abruptly, his demeanor changes. He opens the car door and reaches down to pet Jake's head. Briefly, Jake lays his head in Lannie's lap. Slowly, carefully, he stands. Before he takes the first step, he stops and looks directly into my eyes. I nod affirmatively to him. He raises his fist in salute to the gray sky above and, in a hoarse voice choked with triumphant emotion, says simply, "I made it! I made it!"

Epilogue

Lannie's recovery and subsequent radiation and chemotherapy are another part of the story. If people find this helpful, I plan to write about that as well. Suffice to say that the journey had its joys and challenges. The joys: Our beautiful granddaughter, Audrey, was born January 18—just eight days after Lannie's surgery and just two days after our return home. I was present for her birth, and through a twist of circumstance and fate, Lannie was able to see and hold her just hours after her birth. I had called Lannie as soon as she was born at 3:48 p.m. only to discover that he and Mark were headed to Obici's ED. Lannie's right leg was swelling, and he had to be evaluated for a possible blood clot. I left Alison, Dan, and brand-new little Audrey to meet Lannie and Mark at Obici. Fortunately, the evaluation proved that the swelling was only some excess fluid. Since we were within twenty miles of Alison and our new baby granddaughter, we drove straight to that hospital. They had a wheelchair ready for him, and within minutes, he was holding dear, precious Audrey.

Pain control continued to be a problem, but we eventually conquered it with the help of some wonderful medical and nursing care.

My coworkers continued to be flexible, caring, and supportive so that I could go with Lannie for all his appointments. God also provided for us as he underwent the weeks of radiation treatments (twenty-eight in all). Frank and Judy (Lannies's cousin and husband who were with us for his surgery) had room at their home and welcomed the opportunity to help us. He stayed with them during the week, and Judy drove him every day to his treatments. He came home on weekends. It was hard for me to be separated from him; I missed him painfully. Yet I knew Judy was caring beautifully for him, and I was so grateful. Radiation made him very, very sick. He was extremely nauseated—most likely as a result of the radiation beams going so close to his liver. Again, God blessed us with a wonderful thoracic radiologist and oncologist—Dr. Christopher Kelsey. Dr. Kelsey listened to us, cared about us, and cared for us, and we remain deeply appreciative of him. He was able to prescribe medication to resolve the overwhelming nausea, and at last, Lannie began to improve.

For almost one year, our lives centered around Duke medical appointments and chemotherapy appointments. It was a tough year, and God's grace brought us through. Supportive friends and family made life better. Chemo is as hard as everyone says it is—really tough. Still, we found time and energy to laugh and enjoy our grandchildren and our families. We went on our annual family vacation to Cape Hatteras to the fabulous cottage that Alison had found the preceding November. While vacationing at Cape Hatteras, Lannie felt well enough to fish (his second passion after hunting!) a few days as well.

Our Duke medical team grew to include Dr. Jeffery Crawford and Susan Blackwell, PA. All were caring, knowledgeable, and supportive. Lannie also qualified for a clinical study with Avastin, a chemotherapy agent not yet approved for meso, but definitely worth a try in our opinion. He did very well, all things considered.

Sadly, our dear friend Dave from Matthews County lost his battle with meso in May 2009. His meso came back in his peritoneum, and there wasn't much medicine could do to conquer that. This was a heartbreaking loss for us. Becky and I remain dear friends. She is someone who simply understands because I know she has been there. The bond we share with this generous couple—who so willingly shared their story, love, and support with us when we were so overwhelmed—will always be treasured.

Also, sadly, my dear friends Tracey and Kenneth Stallard (bible verse and comfort basket friend) lost their wonderfully handsome and friendly sixteen-year-old son, Cody, in a tragic car accident less than one mile from their home January 31, 2009. Cody was on his way home from work when the accident occurred. Our wonderful church embraced them with loving care and support. I continue to pray for Kenneth and Tracey.

October 2010 brought bad news to us via a CT scan. Those same lymph nodes seen in his abdomen when his cancer was first discovered and were thought to be safe initially were found to be growing. Eventually, they were biopsied and found to have meso. I took the news very hard. I cried off and on for about three weeks, and then I found my fighting spirit! Just one week after we learned about the cancerous lymph nodes, our beautiful Black Lab, Jake, died from old age. I still miss him.

Lannie underwent another round of five weeks of radiation therapy combined with chemotherapy. His CT scan on June 28, 2011, brought good news of no new spots, and the affected lymph nodes were effectively treated. However, the CT scan on December 13, 2011, showed that two lymph nodes in his abdomen have slightly enlarged. They are in the exact place that the original meso started. Ugh. The doctors tell us the slight enlargement could be just a "normal" response (it is normal for lymph nodes to change slightly in size in response to changes within the body) or it could be the meso making an unwelcome return. They want to simply watch the lymph nodes in questions and rescan in April 2012. This time I remain calmer, more focused as I hear the news. During the three-hour drive back to Ivor, I try to make peace with the fact that it is quite likely that Lannie and I will always be fighting meso on some level. This is our life now. It is a good life. I remain grateful for the progress the medical team has made with treating Lannie and for every moment we have with our family. My thoughts drift to my dear friends Kenneth and Tracey Stallard and their beautiful daughter, Kelly Anne, who daily copes with the chronic illness cystic fibrosis (CF). Many years ago, CF was a deadly disease. As a pediatric nurse, I cared for many children who died from the ravages of this disease. Yet Kelly Anne is a vibrant, healthy looking, absolutely beautiful young woman. Thinking of her fills me with a welcome sense of peace and hope. Yes, I feel fear with the unwelcome news we received regarding the growth of those two lymph nodes. Absolutely. However, I also have faith that God, with His infinite grace, will give us the strength to cope with whatever comes our way.

So what have I learned about faith and fear?

I am certain there is a purpose, a role for fear in our lives. If I didn't fear breast cancer, would I succumb to a yearly mammogram? What about the dreaded colonoscopy? If I didn't fear having a car accident (or being ticketed), would I buckle my seat belt? There is definitely a purpose for fear.

My range of emotions during this experience, as you can tell, ranged from sadness, to grief, to determination and, most importantly, hope. In hindsight, I realize faith was a stabilizer in this turbulent sea of conflicting emotions. I believe that faith can bring each of us as much protection from fear as we allow.

So what else did I learn? At some point in this amazing journey, I began to realize that it is futile for me to try to eliminate the fear associated with Lannie's diagnosis of meso. Fear and worry are common, normal responses to uncertainty. Life with cancer is certainly a breeding ground for fear. I have finally found a measure of peace regarding the dichotomy of fear and faith by recognizing that feeling fear does not mean that I lack faith. I learned that I actively choose to have faith. Faith offers relief from the gnawing, sometimes paralyzing terror that threatens to overwhelm me since cancer made its uninvited intrusion into our lives. Faith is choosing to trust in Him. Faith is believing with certainty that His way is better than anything I know. Faith means that I truly seek and trust God.

I am now able to "feel" faith and describe it—a little. For me, faith is an intriguing combination of hope, positive energy, and wellness. I have learned that faith, for me, is a discipline. It is one I have cultivated through the harrowing experience of fighting my husband's cancer. Like anything cultivated, it continues to change and, hopefully, grow. I am a work in progress.

Lastly, what about cancer? Living with its presence in Lannie is like nothing I ever imagined. Like many others, I sort of thought I had an idea. I didn't. Recently, our grandson, Jackson, provided me with a unique perspective on cancer. He was spending the weekend with us and crawled in bed with me to cuddle, as he often does, early one cool Saturday morning. As he climbed up on our bed to crawl in beside me, he suddenly grabbed his right side and said, "Oh, my side hurts." He looked up at me with a very serious facial expression and said ominously, "I think I have cancer, like Pee-Paw." Intrigued by his statement, I said, "Oh, you do? What is cancer?" He stopped holding his side and sat cross-legged on the bed, looked away momentarily to think for a minute, then looked back at me and said this: "Cancer is what my mommy and I pray about for Pee-Paw every night." I had to smile. As I snuggled his sweet, warm little body next to mine and kissed the top of his little head, I realized how perfect Jackson's simple definition was. Out of the mouths of babes. Yes, cancer is something to be prayed about every moment of each and every day. Yes, I pray cancer will be eradicated. I pray that Lannie's next CT scan will be clear. I pray for strength to help Lannie battle this devastating disease. I give thanks for every day I have with Lannie. I give thanks for good doctors and nurses. I give thanks for a loving family and caring friends. I give thanks for fear. I give thanks for faith.

I pray this story will help someone with Cancer.

I am including some practical information in the form of helpful hints.

Helpful Hints

These are things we learned along the way. Receive them in the spirit we are giving them.

I call them "The Ten Golden Rules" of coping with cancer.

For the Patient and Those Directly Involved (Caretakers)

Dos

1. Be yourself. There are no right or wrong feelings. It is what it is, and you feel what you feel. Absorb the change in your life. Respond accordingly. Your coping method is uniquely yours.

2. Acquire a very complete datebook or organizer to carry with you to all appointments. Get one that also has a pad of paper (legal pad size works well) and pen included. Always have a list of questions ready to ask your doctor. Make sure the organizer zippers shut. Make sure it has both big and little pockets to store your many appointment cards, business cards, prescriptions, and patient reports. Keep this organizer complete and current with your latest questions recorded on your pad of paper so that you can grab it at a moment's notice if you have a sudden appointment.

3. Start a file system for all the bazillion papers you will receive regarding your diagnosis. The Expanda-Files (sold at Target, Wal-Mart, etc.) work well. Start a second file system for the bazillion medical bills you will soon begin receiving. (We did not do this initially, and I sure wish we had!)

4. Have a tote bag packed with comfort items (ChapStick, tissues, ibuprofen, warm socks, a good book, Life Savers, snack foods, a small amount of cash, etc.) that you can grab at a moment's notice. You spend a lot of time in boring, cool waiting rooms. Having a tote filled with comfort items makes the waiting bearable.

5. Maintain an ongoing record of your current medications. Include the name of the medication, the strength, and how often you take it. Post this list in a secure location so that anyone needing it can find it easily.

6. Compose a list of important phone numbers, both electronically (cell phone, computer) and hard copy (paper). Make sure you have those phone numbers readily available at all times. Keep a copy in your organizer. Include family and friends' numbers as well as medical and pharmaceutical numbers.

7. Request a copy of all your medical reports (it is your right as a patient). Include blood work, CT scans, PET scans, pathology reports, etc. Get your own copy of every report. This may save you valuable time if, for some reason, your latest report did not arrive at a specific location. If you are uncomfortable reading your reports, don't read them! Just make sure you can put your hands on them. Make two copies of each. Keep one copy in your organizer for at least six months. File the other one.

8. Research your cancer and find the best medical team for your diagnosis. This may mean that you must travel and leave your comfort zone. Do it! You want the absolute best, most current, reliable care for your kind of cancer. We once met a man in the Duke waiting room who was diagnosed with multiple myeloma. His research showed that the best place to treat him was in Arkansas. So he flew to Arkansas until Duke could really help him. His initial prognosis was grim, and he credits going to

Arkansas as a big part of his success. I found the Internet to be a big help. Yes, I waded through a lot of "stuff," but I also learned a lot helpful information about meso.

9. Establish ground rules regarding information sharing about the cancer diagnosis/prognosis/treatment/progress. Our family chose to be completely honest regarding every aspect of Lannie's journey. Personally, I think honesty is best. Regardless, formulate ground rules regarding information sharing that is agreeable to all the involved parties.

10. Continue to take care of yourself. If you work out regularly, then work out! If you play poker regularly, then play poker! Maintain your friendships. Whatever you do to take care of yourself, continue to do it. You will be healthier and have a better coping ability.

For Friends Who Wish to Support

Dos

1. Go to your friend. Visit frequently. If you can't visit, then call. I will always remember and deeply appreciate our many visitors.

2. Bring food! It doesn't have to be home prepared. Bring a pizza. Bring a rotisserie chicken or fried chicken from a fast-food place. Everything is appreciated. Offer to buy a loaf of bread or a gallon of milk (or toilet paper) if you are at a store. When Lannie was first diagnosed, I was so busy going back and forth to the hospital and then taking him to all the rounds of testing (all while continuing to work full-time) that almost three weeks went by before I made a real grocery trip. Food is really appreciated. After we returned home from Duke following the EPP, our church brought compete meals to us three times a week for a month. I so appreciated that delicious food and the loving thoughtfulness represented in that food. This helped us both recover from the surgery.

3. Give money. I know this sounds crass, but I am being honest. Cancer is a very expensive disease. Parking at a large medical facility usually runs from six to eight dollars per day. In the beginning, gas bills for the car are about three times more than normal as you drive the many rounds for medical testing, consults, etc. Hospital cafeteria food is also very expensive. Overnight stays mean a hotel room as well as the food, gas, etc. Medications and other medical supplies are another huge expense. You can give money tastefully—for example, put a small amount in a greeting card or organize a group donation. If you visit at the hospital, take the family out for a meal and offer to pick up the tab. To be honest, at first, I felt awkward accepting money. However, we really needed it. I remain humbled and so very appreciative

for everyone who helped us. That is the truth. If you can, give money—it is so needed.

4. Offer to do specific chores: mow the grass, provide transportation, vacuum floors, pick up friends/family at the airport, do laundry, empty the garbage, babysit, feed pets, wash dishes, bring mail. One of our dear friends, Susan, mowed our grass and even planted our vegetable garden! She also organized a team to help clean and mulch my flower beds. Lannie loves his vegetable garden, and I love my flowers. I had decided that we would probably have to do without both the vegetable garden and my flower garden the year Lannie was undergoing chemo and radiation. Because of Susan's thoughtfulness, we instead experienced the joy of coming home to colorful flowers and a productive garden thriving in our backyard after a long, exhausting day at Duke. It was a wonderful Welcome Home for us.

5. Avoid the following pitfalls:

Destructive criticizing. If you feel in your heart (and you may be exactly right) that your friend has really made a poor medical choice regarding their doctor or medical facility, find a constructive way to communicate this. Do the legwork involved with a better choice and offer your help. In the end, remember that you have to respect their choice.

Avoid making your friends defend their choices to you.

Avoid complaining to your friend about the stressful situations (like long waits) that they are enduring. You mean well, but no one who has been waiting for hours to be seen needs to hear "You had to wait *how* long to be seen?" or "You drove six hours to see that doctor, and that is *all* that doctor offered you?" Your friend is already enduring the situation, and they don't need to use their energy to listen to you complain about circumstances they have no control over. Instead, offer support. "I know you must be so tired." "I know you must be frustrated." Offer concrete suggestions.

Avoid being a downer.

Avoid being an upper. Be yourself and let your friends be themselves.

6. Be supportive and caring when you visit. *Don't* show up hungry, expecting to be fed or to be hosted when you visit. The family needs you to support them.

7. Be an active listener. People often worry about what to say. That's easy. Say little. Your presence and caring speaks volumes.

8. Be a supportive coworker. Be flexible regarding schedule conflicts. Be understanding regarding sudden schedule changes. Be kind. My coworkers were all these things, and I continue to be appreciative.

9. Continue your support after the initial crisis has passed. Remember, cancer is an ongoing battle. Ask how people are doing. Continue to call and visit. Continue to care.

10. Have fun times with your friend! Laugh! Go to ball games. Go to shows. Go on fishing trips. Go wherever you went to prior to cancer. Laugh more! Joke! Enjoy your friendship.

For Everyone

No matter what, continue to be yourself. Cancer does not define anyone. You are still the same person(s) you have always been. You are *not* cancer. Laugh when you can, cry when you can. Be you!

Index

A

B

C

D

www.ingramcontent.com/pod-product-compliance
Lightning Source LLC
Chambersburg PA
CBHW021237280526
45784CB00005B/2127